MAKING THE ROUNDS

Memoirs of a Small-Town Doctor

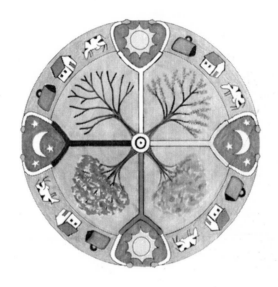

Dr. Gerald L. Miller and Shari Miller Wagner

Published by BookLocker.com, Inc., Bradenton, Florida, U.S.A.

Printed on acid-free paper.

BookLocker.com, Inc.
2015

First Edition .

In Memory of

Dr. Lee Kinzer (1932-2012) and Dr. Victor Binkley (1939-2010)

And for the Staff of the Markle Medical Center

And the Town of Markle, Indiana
Home of 1,102 Happy People and Four Grouches

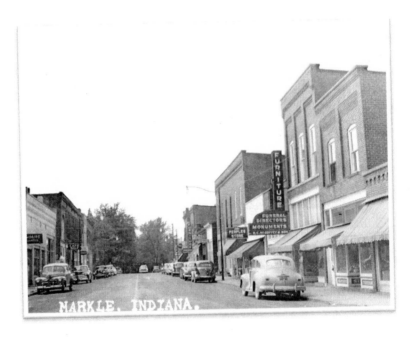

CONTENTS

"A body, love insists, is neither a spirit nor a machine, it is not a picture, a diagram, a chart, a graph, an anatomy; it is not an explanation; it is not a law. It is precisely and uniquely what it is. It belongs to the world of love, which is a world of living creatures, natural orders and cycles, many small, fragile lights in the dark."

—Wendell Berry, from "Health Is Membership"

FOREWORD

The small-town country family doctor. It brings to mind the iconic Norman Rockwell images of the general practitioner of rural America or Dr. Graham, played by Burt Lancaster, in the motion picture *Field of Dreams*. Although romanticized, these characters from the past were actually based on real doctors, and though times have certainly changed, they still exist in some manner today. Many reading this book may fondly remember such a physician who cared for them sometime in their lives.

Small-town docs had the opportunity to experience family medicine to its fullest. They should be considered the quintessential family doctor who practiced their profession in full bloom. They rose early in the morning, went to the hospital to see their patients, and then to their office. They would make house calls sometime during the day, in the evening, or for more urgent needs in the middle of the night. Home deliveries were commonplace, of course, and many family doctors were involved in performing various surgical procedures that would be well beyond the expectations of family physicians today. They generally made themselves unofficially "on duty" twenty-four hours a day, seven days a week. Why? It was because they possessed a sense of responsibility and dedication to their patients and communities that we can only admire and reflect upon today. I believe that at its very core, it was an ever-present desire *to be there* for their patients.

The family doctor was a valued advisor and compassionate counselor who cared for every problem, for everyone in the family from birth to death; the time-honored general practitioner, held in esteem by his or her patients, took the opportunity to talk and develop on-going relationships with patients, advocated for them, and coordinated their health care. These attributes can be validated by anyone who has had a long-term, comforting, and reassuring relationship with their family doc.

The principles and values of family medicine originated during the early and mid-twentieth century, especially among those who ventured out to rural small towns to practice after graduation from medical school or after a year of internship at a hospital. They commonly called themselves general practitioners. In those days, it was not a deprecating term or a term that implied something less than what they were. It was particularly this Greatest Generation of family doctors of mid-century who possessed the character and values which inspired the contemporary formalized specialty of family medicine. Today's family medicine emulates these elder statesmen of general practice from whom it developed and grew.

Now, these core tenets of the discipline of family medicine are incorporated into standardized residency training and board certification. The creation of the American Board of Family Practice in 1969 established family practice as the twentieth medical specialty. The first three-year residency training programs in family practice were established that year.

But no family medicine residency programs existed in those earlier days. The principles of comprehensive and continuous personalized patient care came to the general practitioners of that time by experience and sensitivity to the needs of their patients. They knew their patients well and were committed to their communities. Especially in small towns, they were among the most respected individuals and were considered as trusted friends by their patients. These physicians were humbled and honored to be invited into the lives of their patients.

Family physicians continue to be the heart and soul of medicine. More than any other specialist, family doctors humanize the health-care experience. Focusing their attention on the person, not just the disease, they are driven to develop relationships over generations with the patients and families they care for and by the need to make people whole. Ask any family doc what makes his or her profession rewarding and fulfilling and that's what they will tell you.

But the medical world has changed radically in the last thirty years and continues to rapidly transform. Medicine is fueled by corporate interests and a market-driven health-care system. It is a paradigm that values and promotes procedural medicine and specialty practices maximizing and extracting the most profitable dollars from the health-care system. Primary care physicians are increasingly employed by health-care corporations that judge and pay them mainly on the basis of productivity. Our reimbursement system is not designed to reward spending time with patients to counsel and educate, or to promote health and prevent disease, or to develop the necessary therapeutic relationship by knowing the patient as a person. Medicine is becoming increasingly depersonalized as a system largely dominated by a business ethic. In these contemporary times, family physicians still believe passionately in the traditional values of the specialty, but with these barriers to confront, they're just much more difficult to actualize.

In 2013 I authored the book, *Family Practice Stories* (Indiana Historical Society Press). The book is an oral history of stories told by, or about, forty-eight family doctors who practiced during the mid-twentieth century, mostly in small-town Indiana. The book's goal was to preserve the history and traditions of what many consider to be the Golden Age of Generalism in American medicine, not so much through rote written history but through storytelling. The stories, some serious, some humorous, some sad or touching, are specific episodes in these doctors' careers, mostly taken from original transcripts of the interviews. By reading these stories one can come to know the essence of that era in medicine, appreciate the philosophical underpinnings of family medicine, and also learn countless lessons about character, life, and human values.

I was pleased to be asked to write the foreword to *Making the Rounds*. As I read its chapters, I was taken with how much this book and my own complement each other. Both carry you to a different period, a simpler and more personal time, a time when professionalism, the art of medicine, and the art of healing were at a zenith. I was struck by the emergence of the same lessons, values, and themes, but this time, in *Making the Rounds*, through the career of a single physician, Gerald Miller.

Dr. Miller was much like the many family doctors in *Family Practice Stories*, including my own father, a general practitioner in South Bend, Indiana for forty years. They were all cut from the same fabric. A lifelong Hoosier, Dr. Miller graduated from Indiana University School of

Medicine in 1963 and completed a one-year internship at Lutheran Hospital in Fort Wayne, Indiana. He and his good friend and medical school classmate, Lee Kinzer, were recruited by the townspeople of Markle, Indiana after being approached by the widow of the doctor who had served that community for many years. There was a compelling, community need for a couple of family doctors, and they were warmly welcomed with kindness and gratitude into the community in which they eventually served for over four decades.

Like many small-town docs, Dr. Miller became integrated into the community in many ways. He taught Sunday school and served as deacon at his church; he served on the school board and established the local hospice program; he served as the medical director for a local nursing home and a retirement center; he became the chairman of the board of the State Bank of Markle and also his local hospital. He was the sideline physician during high school football games, established the region's emergency medical services organization, volunteered with the Lion's Club, and won recognition from his community with many awards. He understood, typical of small-town physicians, that there was much more to assuring the health and wellbeing of his community than purely the provision of medical care within the walls of the exam room.

I recall my father frequently telling us at the dinner table about a patient he had seen that day in his office. The story was not so much about the medical aspects of the patient but about something interesting the patient had told him. It could have been about family members, an event, an unusual situation, or just something about his or her life. I suspect that Dr. Miller did the same.

Today, we hear a lot about "mindfulness," the ability or, probably more accurately, the willingness, to take notice and appreciate the details of your immediate world and to care for the present moment. Many family doctors listened attentively to their patients and absorbed themselves in their patients' stories during an office visit. When the exam door closed, the world was limited to that small space and their attention was focused on the patient, not only their medical issues, but even the small details of their life stories. Listening is a common theme in the stories in my book and the book you are reading. This attribute was one of the essential foundations upon which these doctors built lasting personal relationships with their patients. Ultimately, these relationships are the greatest reward family physicians receive in their career.

As you read this book you will begin to notice that the stories that Dr. Miller relates aren't only about him and his medical practice. His personal story intertwines with the stories of his patients and comes to blend with the history and the story of the community. They become one story. It is a natural destination, as the authors acknowledge he understood that he was part of something important and bigger than himself. I found that so many of the small town family physicians of that era express that very belief. There is a remarkable commonality of emotion and experience manifested by these physicians as they reflect on what their patients and communities meant to them during this extraordinary time.

There is an old saying that what you do for yourself dies with you, but what you do for others lives on. That typifies the small-town family doc. That characterizes Dr. Gerald Miller.

This book is described by the authors as a love letter to the people of Markle. Dr. Miller touched the lives of his patients and community, and his patients and community touched his heart in return. It is a beautiful story of a family doctor committed to the rural Indiana town he called home.

Yes, a love letter. I like that.

Richard Feldman, M.D., FAAFP
Director of Medical Education and Family Medicine
Residency Training, Franciscan St. Francis Health,
Indianapolis
Former Indiana State Health Commissioner
April, 2015

PREFACE

*M*aking the Rounds is the second book my father and I have written together. Our first collaboration, *A Hundred Camels: A Mission Doctor's Sojourn and Murder Trial in Somalia*, fulfilled a promise I penned in my eighth-grade journal—that one day I would write a book about my father's murder trial, a frightening event and no less absurd to me than the court scene from *Alice's Adventures in Wonderland*. As it turned out, my father harbored a strong desire to tell that story, too—a story that included the tenacity of a Somali family who knew he was innocent and refused to accept the court's verdict and the payment of blood money. Thirty-five years after we left Somalia, Dad and I began a book that became much more than an account of a murder trial and more than a story about the challenges faced by an Indiana doctor practicing tropical medicine in a remote Somali village. *A Hundred Camels* evolved into our collaborative love letter to an ancient Islamic land rich in terms of folklore and proverbs, affluent in terms of hospitality, friendship, and traditions of faith.

A year after *A Hundred Camels* was published, Dad and I started another book—the one you are holding. *Making the Rounds: Memoirs of a Small-Town Doctor* recounts my father's life work as a family doctor practicing medicine in the last half of the twentieth-century. But it is also our love letter to a particular place and its people—this time the rural town of Markle, Indiana. This small town is a predominately white, Protestant community, eight thousand miles from the Somali village of Jamama, yet it is similarly wealthy in terms of history and folklore and well-to-do in relation to generosity, friendship, and sense of community. In 1964, this town raised money to help my dad and his medical partner, Lee Kinzer, set up their practice, and a few years later it sent a petition to President Johnson requesting that the doctors remain in Markle during the Vietnam War. I was lucky to grow up in this remarkable community—to swim in its quarry, coast my bike down its hill, and watch its ballgames and Wildcat Parades.

My father brought forty-two years of stories, experience, and wisdom to this project, while I contributed my skills as a writer and researcher. For almost all of these chapters, Dad wrote the first drafts and then I set to work crafting the prose and adding descriptive and historical details, quotations, and any additional information I gleaned from our weekly lunch dates and frequent phone calls and emails. The result, we believe, is a collaboration that reaches deeper and tells a story more accurately than if either one of us had written it alone.

One of our foremost hopes is that *Making the Rounds* illustrates how essential it is for doctors to take adequate time to listen to their patients. When my father looks back, he says that the main reason he enjoyed his medical practice so much was because he was listening to stories. He didn't enter his profession with the expectation of that reward, but he did assume he would do a great deal of listening. His teachers at Indiana University School of Medicine made sure he knew that. They underscored the importance of understanding a patient's story and then performing a complete and thorough physical exam. Dad learned that the ability to listen and ask the right questions is no less important to a doctor than skills in science and math. The stories he heard on his hospital rounds, in the office, and on house calls helped him to form patient histories, make diagnoses, and avoid ordering unnecessary tests.

But my father didn't just listen to stories related to illness. He asked patients about their daily lives and what was happening in their families. What he heard reminded him that he was not just treating diseases but attending to people—unique individuals connected to a family and community. He especially enjoyed house calls to older patients who might give him descriptions of folk remedies or anecdotes about previous town doctors or what it was like when Markle's brass band played on Morse Street every Wednesday night. Their vivid memories connected him to his landscape and earlier generations of townsfolk and farmers.

My father and I hope this book reveals the main advantage of living in a small town or rural community—the sense of belonging it offers. In his essay, "Health Is Membership," Wendell Berry traces the word *health* back to its Indo-European root as *heal* and *whole* and argues that, as a standard of health, communal wholeness— "the sense of belonging to others and a place"—is as important as individual wholeness. But this benefit of small-town communities is often overlooked, especially by those driving through on a street turned into a highway where yards are shaved off to make a quicker route. Too many towns in Indiana and elsewhere have main streets where store buildings stand empty or have been converted into living quarters. In many such towns, the most successful businesses are the antique shops that profit from the past. In Indiana, alone, there are four hundred and forty cities and towns with populations of fewer than five thousand. Many of these communities have trouble attracting young people, and high school graduates who go off to college like me seldom come back. As a result, doctors and other professionals tend to be scarce. A hard fact is that only ten percent of U.S. physicians live in rural areas, but they serve twenty-five percent of the nation's population.

Obsessed with technology, our society speaks of the body as if it were a machine. But it's not. It's a living, natural thing that belongs in a community. Maybe my father's upbringing in a Mennonite community and my early years in Markle predispose us to believe that. Yet it just makes good sense that people are healthier when they feel connected to each other and the place where they live. Dad was an active member of his community, treating patients but also standing along the sidelines of football games, selling brooms door to door, balancing on the hot seat of a dunk tank, racing with an outhouse, and sitting on the school board and bank board.

Late at night, when he drove on house calls, he was alone in his car but still at the heart of something larger. His headlight beams were not the only lights in the darkness. It was a familiar countryside illuminated by moon, stars, and fireflies, by porch lights of old farm houses, and the security lights of small towns.

Shari Miller Wagner

ACKNOWLEDGMENTS

First of all, the authors wish to thank Tamara Dubin Brown (see https://suburbansatsangs.wordpress.com/), artist and writer, for the original artwork on the book cover. Her design adopts traditional elements of the Native American medicine wheel (cardinal directions and colors) as it celebrates the rounds of a family doctor and the relationship between community membership and health. Sydney Brown (see www.facebook.com/sydneybrownart), illustrator and design artist, provided much-appreciated technical expertise in the reproduction of the photographs inside this book.

The authors gratefully acknowledge all those who gave feedback on the book's content. This includes Iona Wagner who carefully proofread and commented on the entire manuscript, as well as those who shared responses to earlier versions or individual chapters: Ryan Ahlgrim, John Bender, Marty Bender, J. Daniel Hess, Amee Hofstetler, John Hofstetler, Martha Yoder Maust, M.D., Paul Shankland, Catherine Swanson, Julianna Thibodeaux, and Chuck Wagner.

Additionally, they want to express deep appreciation to the people of the Markle community who contributed to this project. The photographs of Morse Street and the Thomas Mill are provided courtesy of Gary Girvin and Rob and Debbie Randol. Janice Jordan, Marlene Hoopingarner, Linda Reed, and Janice Spahr shared their memories from working at the Markle Medical Center. Patricia Fuller graciously allowed the authors to include her late husband's previously unpublished account of his near-death experience. Jerry and

Jean Mossburg took the authors on a field trip back in time to find the remains of the old Rock Creek mill and the clearing where the Miami once held their dances.

Finally, the authors are especially grateful to Mary Miller for her assistance in recalling past events and for collecting local source material, especially previous issues of the *Markle Times*. This monthly newspaper is a treasure trove of historical information about Markle, and the authors wish to convey their abiding gratitude to Mary and other editors and writers of that valuable publication.

INTRODUCTION

My father has gone on rounds for most of his life. As a boy growing up in the Mennonite community of Shipshewana, Indiana, those rounds took the form of farm chores—every evening he fed the calves, milked the cows, cleaned the milking equipment, forked manure, and then threw hay and straw from the loft. In high school the rounds increased. After classes each day, he worked as the school's second-floor janitor—emptying wastebaskets, sweeping floors, and cleaning commodes. As a full-time college student, with a wife and child to support, he managed a complicated round of weekly activities that included, among other things, attending classes, doing homework, washing bakery trucks, and waiting on department store customers. Of course, as a medical student and intern, he made hospital rounds—sometimes the same rounds twice in one morning—once by himself and then with a supervising clinician.

After he and his medical partner, Lee Kinzer, set up their practice south of Fort Wayne in Markle, my father made rounds at three hospitals, sometimes two or even three times a day. Eventually, he narrowed the rounds to just the Wells Community Hospital, but there were still rounds of house calls and night calls, office appointments, nursing home and hospice visits; rounds to see patients in jail; rounds of football games as team physician; rounds of monthly schoolboard meetings and bank board meetings; the annual door-to-door rounds of collecting donations for the Lion's Club eye bank, the rounds of the annual town parade he watched or walked or rode in; the rounds of Sunday school and EMT classes he taught; the perpetual rounds of babies to deliver and funerals to attend; the turning of the seasons he saw from his car as he drove all over two rural counties, year round.

I could recall more rounds, but I'm already dizzy. I don't know how he did so much, and he says he doesn't either, though he figures it had something to do with the fact that he was well-organized. It helped to have a certain routine to follow—a given order to the farm chores and later to office and hospital visits.

But how did he do so much and yet never appear to be rushed? How did he find time to converse with his patients about their children, hobbies, favorite sports teams, or long ago memories of Markle, while he knew there was still much he needed to get around to doing? How could he always appear so calm and rooted to the present moment?

Of course, my father is only one of many amazing family doctors of his generation and earlier who took ample time with their patients while juggling rounds of patient visits and community activities. Dr. Kinzer made lots of house calls and also found time to play on a softball league, participate in his Methodist church, and raise six children. My father's predecessor, Dr. Haldon Woods, had no medical partner, and yet, despite daytime and evening office hours, he'd drop by a patient's house just for a cup of coffee or maybe to leave a gallon of his home-made Elixir of Rhubarb.

At the risk of being charged with circular reasoning, I'd like to propose that perhaps this immense energy had something to do with all of the rounds—all of those rounds making these doctors part of a circle. After all, it's the wheel that moves bikes, cars, and trains and the sphere of our earth that carries us through space. "My business is circumference," the poet Emily Dickinson once wrote. That's also the business of family doctors. As they go on their rounds, they're an integral part of their community circle. There must be something invigorating in that—belonging to something bigger than themselves, serving others through illness and wellness, being present for the first cries of birth and the last words before death.

It seems fitting that this book does not always move by chronology, but sometimes leaps forward and back as if time itself were a circle, with past and present joined together. Indeed, circles are at the heart of this book. When you live in a place like Markle, you're a part of so many circles: circles of friendship and reciprocity and shared stories. Markle, with its intersecting river, roads, and train tracks, has traditionally been a hub for the surrounding rural community—and in this book, too, it serves as the hub—the pivot—the core.

A Miami village once stood at the confluence of Rock Creek and the Wabash. Markle residents can still locate the dance ground. Native Americans whose villages have stood where many of our towns now stand have known that circumference is part of the healing process. Their medicine wheels symbolize wholeness, of being at the center of something larger than yourself and reaching out in all directions.

Shari Miller Wagner

ONE: AN OPEN DOOR

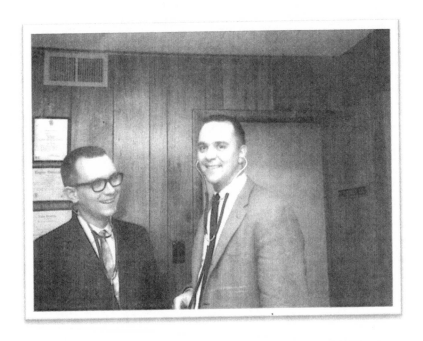

THE SEARCH

For the most part, I appreciated my late night drives to and from house calls or the hospital. The rural roads were mostly empty, and I had time to think over my day or the next day's schedule. Sometimes I just enjoyed the way the cornfields looked in the moonlight and the solitary dignity of Hoosier farmhouses and barns. Sometimes I thought about the small towns I passed—many of them almost ghost towns with names that intrigued me: *Plum Tree, Buckeye, Browns Corner, Banner City, Rockford, Rock Creek Center, Simpson,* and *Mardenis.* Almost in an eye blink, I could drive by these hamlets, but I wondered what they were like in their heyday—before railroad companies pulled up their tracks or gasoline companies abandoned their wells or highways diverted customers to the cities.

Fortunately, some folks remembered. Patients near Mardenis told me the town once had a railroad station and a hotel that attracted gamblers from Chicago. Plum Tree was called Yankeetown until a tree bearing plums grew from a branch a farmer stuck in the mud. The farmer had been using the branch as a switch to drive his stubborn cow. At night, I mused on such towns that slipped past in the darkness, with maybe only a security light or porch light for a marker.

Sometimes, though, as I drove home, I had trouble staying awake. Then I would search for an FM station or whistle the tune of a folksong or hymn. If that didn't work, a certain story would shake me awake: the memory of how my predecessor, Dr. Haldon Woods, vanished one night while driving home from the hospital.

7

I was an intern when I first heard the story of the doctor's disappearance. It was a day that determined the course of my life. I had finished my morning rounds and was about to enter my pathology class when the instructor, Dr. Griest, put his hand on my shoulder. "Wait, Gerald," he said, stopping me outside the door. He had already pulled aside Lee Kinzer, another intern.

"I'd like you both to go down to the front lounge," the pathologist said. "You'll find two ladies who would like to speak to an intern. One of them is a Mrs. Woods. Don't worry about missing my lecture." Then, without waiting for a response, the doctor turned and entered his classroom.

Lee and I exchanged a quizzical glance. "Do you know what this is about?" I asked as we walked toward the elevator.

"Dr. Griest asked me if we're still thinking about going into practice together," Lee said, "so I figure this has something to do with that."

It was mid-November 1963, and both of us were fulfilling a year of post-grad medical training at Fort Wayne's Lutheran Hospital. Our friendship had developed a few years earlier, during medical school in Indianapolis, when we both attended the local chapter of the Christian Medical Society. Lee sported a flattop like I did, but he was taller—a few inches over six feet—and six years older. He had been drafted straight out of high school as a pitcher by the St. Louis Cardinals but after a year in the minors injured his back sliding into home plate. The doctor prescribed two weeks in bed, a year and a half in a back brace, and no more baseball.

If Lee couldn't play professional sports, he still liked talking about them. As we waited for the elevator, he brought up a recent Steeler-Redskin game. "Did you see Ballman's ninety-two-yard kickoff return?" Lee asked. He was a big Pittsburgh fan, while I rooted for the Bears.

"I heard about it, but I was watching Chicago," I said and left it at that since Lombardi's Packers had pounded my Bears, 27 to 7.

Lee grinned. "That must have been an exciting game." Just then the elevator arrived. On the way down he added, "Next Sunday we'll see how your Willie Galimore stacks up against John Henry Johnson."

The door opened, and we entered the lounge, empty except for two women who stopped speaking to glance over at us.

"We're here to meet a Mrs. Woods," Lee said as we approached.

"That's me," replied the younger of the two, a petite, middle-aged woman, dark-haired, and dressed in a jacket and skirt. "I'm Mary Ellen, and this is Mrs. Etta Heaston." She motioned towards a kind-faced woman with short, curly red hair. "Etta was my husband's receptionist."

We all shook hands, and then Mrs. Woods suggested we sit down. "I'm here because my town needs a doctor," she said, earnestly.

"What town is that?" I asked.

"Markle. It's about a half hour south of here."

"I know that town. I've driven through there," Lee said. "I went to college at Taylor, and Markle is about thirty miles north."

I tried to read from Lee's amiable tone and expression his opinion of Markle, but I couldn't tell.

"Haldon, my husband, was the town's only physician for twenty-four years," Mrs. Woods continued. "The only time he left was to serve in WWII, and when he came back, he was busier than ever, driving to several hospitals each day and keeping daytime and evening office hours." She went on to say that when her husband developed insulin-dependent diabetes, these long hours became especially hard on him.

"Late one night, about a year ago, he left home to see a patient at Huntington Hospital and never returned," Mrs Woods said. "I thought maybe he decided to just spend the night at the hospital, but in the morning when I phoned, the nurse told me he left for home at about 2 a.m., soon after he arrived."

When she learned that her husband's cream-colored sedan was last seen heading north out of Huntington, Mrs. Woods presumed he was driving to Warsaw where he occasionally went to relax at Winona Lake, only about forty miles away. But after several days passed and he still hadn't returned, she notified the Sheriff's Department. Police searched the gravel pits and wooded areas in Huntington County but discovered no clues. Tips started coming in from people who said they saw the doctor in Indianapolis or on a Chicago street, strolling with an unknown woman. One person speculated he was hiding in Ohio because of tax evasion charges.

"We found out the truth three weeks later," Mrs. Woods said.

One of her husband's patients, Charles Scott, woke up from a dream in which he saw the doctor's car miss the curve at the Henrick farm. The next day, Charles told his friend Max Becker about this disturbing dream as they drove to work. On their way home, they decided to check it out. It was hard to see where the car left State Route 224. There weren't any skid marks because of the curve, but they were able to follow tire tracks through the cornfield and into a ravine.

There, crashed against a tree, was the doctor's car.

After missing the curve the sedan apparently cut through the field's edge for a few hundred feet and then plummeted into the gully where it hit the tree head-on. An autopsy revealed that the forty-eight year-old doctor died on impact. He either fell asleep while driving or blacked out because of an insulin reaction.

Mrs. Woods shook her head and gazed at the gray carpet. "Haldon was only two miles from Markle, almost home."

"Dr. Woods was a wonderful doctor," Mrs. Heaston said. "We all miss him so much."

"Now we desperately need another doctor," Mrs. Woods said, looking at us. "For a year I've been getting phone calls, all with the same question, 'Can you direct me to a doctor?' But most of the doctors in the surrounding towns aren't taking new patients. My husband's patients have either gone without a physician or driven far from home to receive help. Finally, the idea came to me—to come here to the hospital and ask for a doctor just starting out. I'd be willing to sell my husband's office for a very reasonable sum.

It has all the furniture and equipment. Everything looks just as it did on his last day."

"But would there be enough work for two doctors?" Lee asked. "Gerald and I are planning to go into practice together."

"I'm sure there would be," Mrs. Woods said. "I wish Haldon had taken a partner to ease his workload. I was surprised when both of you walked in, but I'm certain there would be enough work."

"How many people live in Markle? I asked.

"About eight hundred," Mrs. Heaston replied.

That didn't sound all that small to me since my hometown was less than half that size.

"You would also see many farmers and some patients from surrounding towns," Mrs. Woods added. "It's a good place to raise a family. People look out for each other."

We asked a few more questions, but then it was time for me to give new patients their physicals and Lee to work an emergency room shift. Before excusing ourselves, we assured the two women that we were definitely interested and would be happy to meet with the search committee the townsfolk had formed.

As we waited for elevators to take us in separate directions, I asked Lee what Markle was like.

"The downtown doesn't look like much, but there's a park that caught my attention. It's right before you cross the Wabash, coming from the south. There's a pool made from a quarry and a softball field much nicer than you see in most small towns. It's got lights with a concession stand and bleachers."

I asked if he remembered anything else.

"A scoreboard and an announcer's booth," Lee joked. "No, seriously, there isn't much to see—a few stores, two grain elevators, and some houses."

We agreed that we were impressed by Mrs. Woods and her determination to find a doctor. We were also curious to learn more about a town where a doctor's car could swerve into his patient's dream. Then Lee's elevator door slid open and so did mine.

For the rest of the day, between patients, my thoughts kept returning to Markle. I wondered if this might be the opportunity Lee and I had been hoping for. Dr. Gentile, a doctor we both liked, had recently asked us to join his established practice, but we hadn't given him an answer yet. Neither of us wanted to live in Fort Wayne. Lee's wife, Dawn, and my wife, Mary, weren't keen on living there, either—or, for that matter, in any large city. Lee grew up in Pittsburgh and wanted to experience life in a small town. Mary and I had lived on farms near Shipshewana, Indiana and hoped a door to some similar community would swing open.

Maybe this was that door.

SHIPSHEWANA

Shipshewana was named for a Potawatomi chief whose name meant "Vision of a Cougar." He also had an English name—Peter the Great—given to him by the French priest who baptized him. Although the Potawatomi converted to Christianity, that didn't deter white farmers from wanting their fertile land. More than eight hundred and fifty Potawatomi, including Chief Shipshewana, were pushed at gun and bayonet point from Northern Indiana to Osawatomie, Kansas in the autumn of 1838. The six-hundred-and-sixty-mile journey took sixty-one days and has been called "The Potawatomi Trail of Death." Along the way, forty people, mostly children, died of typhoid fever and the stress of a forced march through thick dust and unseasonable heat.

Soon after Chief Shipshewana reached the Kansas reservation, he slipped back to Indiana, traveling by night. There, after finding the burnt remains of his village on the shore of what is now Shipshewana Lake, he lived in the marshes. Two years later, he was buried in an unmarked grave. I have sometimes wondered why the chief didn't stay in Kansas with his people. Most likely, he considered his community as encompassing more than just people—it included the land and its creatures, the graves of his ancestors, and the stories that connected him in a tangible way to the past and the present.

I was born almost a hundred years after the Potawatomi Removal. As I was growing up, my hometown had only about three hundred residents, but it was the center of an expansive Mennonite and Amish agricultural community.

The town's tallest structure was a grain elevator, and its business district also included a stockyard, lumberyard, two grocery stores, a dry goods store, a bank, pharmacy, and three diners. Entertainment venues were scarce, no movie theatres or bowling alleys or dance halls, but there was a summer activities program at the school, swimming at Shipshewana Lake, and many social activities sponsored by my church—Forks Mennonite.

During my boyhood summers, I worked half days in the fragrant mint fields, thinning and transplanting plants. Later, when the peppermint was harvested, it would be boiled down in a vat and made into peppermint oil to flavor gum and candies. My family sometimes used a few drops of peppermint oil in the nose as a decongestant; my wife's family sprinkled drops on their handkerchiefs to unplug a nose and soothe the soreness from blowing. I remember Mary's grandfather, George Dintaman, used it so liberally on his arthritic joints that he always smelled slightly of mint.

Once I reached high school age, I painted houses and barns with my father, Perry, a history teacher and the principal of Shipshewana School. Each summer my dad hired a painting crew of teachers, as well as high school and college students. He had a penchant for singing "Nearer My God to Thee" as he balanced on the highest rungs of a ladder, painting the peak of a barn. We had to watch out for curious livestock that might bump against our propped ladders. Sometimes for additional height we perched ladders on top of farm wagons and then used rocks to hold the wheels in place. But no matter how tightly we wedged the stones, a hog could still jiggle a tilted ladder while it used the adjacent wheel as a scratching post.

One of the things I liked best about living on a farm was that I could work with animals. At the age of nine I joined 4-H and cared for a Guernsey heifer calf as my project. Each year I bought another calf and showed her in local and state competitions. By my senior year I owned a small dairy herd that I sold to buy a car and help pay for my college expenses. I also enjoyed helping my father with his cows and would sometimes tend a farmer's orphaned lamb or raise a dozen chicks from the local hatchery. Besides feeding my chickens, I had to keep a look-out for the turkey buzzards that would glide over the farmyard searching for pullets.

One August evening, just after my eleventh birthday, I was milking Betsy, our oldest cow, when I heard a tremendous thunder crack and saw a simultaneous flash. Betsy staggered. The lights went out. The motor on the Globe milking machine sputtered to a stop and started smoking. My first thought was that now I'd be milking all four cows by hand. When I ran to the atrium of the barn, I could see smoke puffing from a light bulb socket and the hay mow. I started up the ladder with a bucket of water and near the top spotted the flames.

My parents were at a district church meeting, so I was home alone with my two sisters, thirteen-year-old Jewel and three-year-old Sally Jo. I unfastened Betsy and the other cows from their stanchions, shooed them from the barn, and led the penned calves outside. By then, thick smoke was everywhere. I ran to the house door to tell Jewel to call the fire department, but she soon yelled back that the phone line was dead. She sped on her bike to the neighbors west of us, while I pedaled as hard as I could toward our neighbors to the east. On my way back, I heard the Shipshewana fire alarm sounding and saw flames shooting from the barn roof. When I reached home, Sally Jo stood in the yard, crying.

Within a day news had spread that the Miller family had lost their barn and everything in it but the cows. Farmers arrived with their trucks and tractors to clean up the charred site. A neighbor offered us the use of an empty barn where we could shelter and milk our cows. A number of farmers, including the Amish, gave us free hay, straw, and feed. One farmer donated trees from his woods that a portable sawmill cut into lumber for the frame and beams of our new barn. I saw firsthand how a community came together when a neighbor was in need. Later, I missed that sense of community in Indianapolis and Fort Wayne. People along King Street in Indy kept moving, often to the suburbs, and though Mary and I lived there four years, we only knew two of our neighbors. In Fort Wayne our only friends were other interns and their families.

That new barn was better than the old one; it had a cement floor, a separate attached milk house, and a modern milking parlor that enabled us to sell grade-A milk and use a new Surge milking machine. It also boasted a hip roof with a top floor that was smooth and solid. From what would ordinarily be just a hay mow, my dad designed a full basketball court with a hoop at each end and good lighting. My friends and I spent many nights up there shooting and dribbling—perfecting our basketball skills. After all, this was Indiana in the 40s and 50s, when high school teams generated more excitement than IU and Purdue. I played guard for the Shipshe Indians and learned the importance of teamwork in the era of Bobby Plump, Oscar and Bailey Robertson, and Jimmy Rayl.

After the meeting with Mrs. Woods, Mary and I wondered how much Markle was like Shipshe. We knew it wouldn't be a Mennonite and Amish community. Even from a road map, the town looked more "worldly." Shipshewana had only one line passing through it, the straight, thin line of Road 5, while Markle had lots of intersecting lines: the wavy blue one of the river, a dotted county line, and the routes of three highways.

THE INTERVIEW

Sometimes, in retrospect, you see a pattern in unrelated events—a synchronicity you never noticed earlier. During the course of one November week, I thought about two men I had never known personally, both in their forties when they died. They served in WW II, worked hard, sacrificed their time for others, and, when they died, left behind wives who persevered with dignity. One was mourned by his small-town community. Another, by his nation.

I was driving my '55 Chevy with the radio on when I learned that President John F. Kennedy had been shot. Mary was ironing in the living room and watching *As the World Turns*. The moment the news broke seems suspended now. The Singing Nun is cut-off in the midst of "Dominique." Mary's soap opera is interrupted and her ironing, forgotten. Of course, after the shock time moved on. It always does. In the Midwest, the last leaves of one November drift into the yard of the next.

After a Thanksgiving I spent on call at the hospital, arrangements were made for a late afternoon interview in Markle. When the day arrived, Lee drove since he was familiar with the route. We talked about questions the search committee might ask as we passed the town of Zanesville and then empty cornfields and scattered farm houses with barns. Eventually, the houses started appearing closer together and in the distance I noticed the tall storage bins of a grain elevator.

"We're a bit early," Lee said as we drove by the elevator and over a double set of train tracks. "Let's turn at the intersection and see what's along 224. I haven't driven along that stretch."

Going east, we passed by the front of the Agrarian Grain elevator, a Veterans of Foreign Wars building, several houses, and then the Slumber Inn—a modest Mom-and-Pop motel. Heading west, we saw a few blocks of small wooden houses, the town cemetery, and the limestone edifice of Markle Church of the Brethren. I was pleased to see a Church of the Brethren, a denomination with tenets similar to Mennonites: belief in adult baptism, nonviolence, and service to others.

"It gets better," Lee said as we turned around in the cemetery and headed back past houses set much too close to the highway. I hoped that by spring this part of the town would appear more cheerful. Now, nothing, not even a light dusting of early December snow, softened the stark tree branches and houses, and a gray sky compounded the melancholy.

When we turned back onto Road 3 (Clark Street), I was relieved to see that the town did become more attractive. Freed from the highway, the yards were more spacious and the houses, older and larger, had side yards and porches. This street sloped downhill toward the Wabash River and the business district. We passed a grocery, two barber shops, a garage, and an A&W drive-in before turning left onto Morse, the town's main street. After driving by a block of brick storefronts, we parked near a tall, wooden thermometer staked in the bank's front yard. Silver paint indicated that the town had almost reached its goal of four thousand dollars for the doctor's fund. Later, we learned it raised more than six thousand dollars, all of it earmarked to help purchase Dr. Woods' office building and equipment.

Lee and I expected to be interviewed by members of the search committee, but the bank's conference room was packed with business leaders, farmers, young parents, and retirees, each prepared to let us know the town needed a doctor.

I was particularly touched by the words of one elderly man, Freeman Truby, who stood up to speak with a voice wavering from age and emotion: "My wife, Alice, and I have been praying every night for a doctor to come to Markle, and now my prayers are being answered."

Several people said they knew we would be busy right away since most of Dr. Woods' patients hadn't seen a doctor since his death. Only a few expressed concern as to whether there would be enough business for two doctors.

At the end of the meeting, the search committee escorted us across the street to see Dr. Woods' office, a building with *Woods* stenciled on the window in white lettering. To the east stood Reed's Television, and to the west, the storeroom for a furniture store. The doctor's office was narrow and squat compared to most of the buildings on Morse Street, but when the florescent lights flickered on, we discovered it was unusually long. Behind the front waiting area where worn chairs lined the walls and end tables displayed past issues of magazines, we found two small examining rooms, their white enamel cabinets stocked with hemostats, surgical scissors, and speculums. Glass jars contained cotton balls or stood empty, their alcohol gone dry.

Across the hallway, shelves in a narrow drug dispensary stored gallon jugs of cough medicine and dusty bottles of antacids, aspirin, and other pills, some with dates that still had not expired. Though it was obvious that Dr. Woods dispensed much of the medicine he prescribed, I asked if there was a pharmacy in town. The nearest, I was told, was about ten miles away in Huntington.

Beyond the pharmacy and a small restroom was a workroom with a door to the alley and gravel parking area. This workroom, with its Bunsen burner, test tubes, and centrifuge for spinning down urine samples, was equipped for simple lab tests. Crossing the hall, we entered a smaller room where the nurse had kept track of patient care on 4 x 6 index cards that documented the date of each office visit and gave a brief description of treatment, usually just a line.

This building was small for one doctor and could never accommodate two. Most buildings along Morse Street sported a second story and, some, even a third, but this structure had only the ground floor and a small unfinished basement, dim and damp. A closet beneath the staircase harbored a real human skeleton, and a shelf with glass jars of formaldehyde held fetuses in advancing stages of development. Lined up on more shelves, a dozen or more two-gallon bottles labeled "Dr. Woods' Elixir of Rhubarb" stockpiled enough laxative for a whole county, I estimated— sufficient to last two years, if so needed.

When I asked about the possibility of more office space, a committee member told us that the three elderly sisters who owned the furniture storeroom had indicated they might be willing to sell.

Before we left that night we also asked about the schools. Lee and Dawn had four young children—Mark, Mike, Leah, and Matt—and Mary and I had five-year-old

Shari and two-year-old Marlis. We learned that until 1956 Markle had its own school with twelve grades, but now, because the town was split by four townships, students attended four different township schools. Prevailing thought was that soon, with consolidation efforts underway, each county would have only one or two high schools.

Markle did have its own half-day kindergarten run by the local Psi Iota Xi sorority and held in the former Veterans of Foreign Wars building. A young banker who was with us—Don Hoopingarner—said that if we moved to town Shari would finish her year of kindergarten with his own daughter, Pam.

Markle encompassed five churches and a community park with a softball diamond, playground, swimming pool, and a scout cabin half-hidden in the woods. It possessed a steep hill children could coast bikes down and a river—the Wabash—that meandered past the bottom of that hill, behind Morse Street. The Old Thomas Mill still ground flour at the Markle Dam, and the Erie Lackawana rail line still stretched across the north side of town and retained a working station.

Driving back, Lee and I compared notes. We had both been deeply moved by the words of Mr. Truby and also impressed by those of Bill Randol, the local barber, who said he not only wanted good health care for his wife and three children, but also for his extended family, which included the Duncans, Suttons, Allreds, and Highlands. Farmers had attended the meeting, too, an indication that those living outside of town were searching for a doctor. We naturally appreciated the warm and generous spirit that was raising the mercury in the bank yard thermometer. All in all, it seemed a rare and wonderful thing to find a community so willing to help new doctors set up a practice.

SETTING UP

Markle seemed like what Mary and I and the Kinzers had been hoping for—a small town where medical care was needed and our families could join a vibrant community. Our decision to come was an easy one, but after that the choices grew harder.

After years of studying the facts of healthcare and how to apply them to the needs of patients, Lee and I faced the sudden challenge of setting up a practice, an endeavor essentially the same as starting a small business. Fortunately, our internship program dictated that every other Friday afternoon we visit a different medical office to see patients and talk with physicians about how they organized their practices. We knew how to remove warts and earwax, stitch cuts, and stop nosebleeds, but how would we decide what fees to charge, what appointment system to use, how many nurses to hire, how to file insurance? We received answers to some of those questions, but many doctors did not want to share financial information with other physicians. And then, of course, there were many important questions we didn't know to ask.

One of our first challenges to tackle was hiring our staff. Initially, our wives would help out since years of education-related expenses had left us financially strapped. Fortunately, neither family had accumulated much debt. During Lee's medical school years, Dawn had worked as a registered nurse. My parents assisted us by purchasing a small, red-brick bungalow near the IU campus in Indianapolis where we lived rent free, and Mary's folks kept our freezer full of meat and vegetables from their farm. For all four years, Mary and I earned money by selling lecture notes to my two hundred classmates. I took notes and hired a couple of other students to take them, too. After I compiled and formatted these reports, Mary typed them on a portable typewriter with mimeograph paper, using a razor blade to scrape off mistakes. She still calls this job a nightmare as it involved deciphering medical terms from my poor handwriting.

Now Mary was willing to use her bookkeeping and receptionist skills at the new office, and Dawn volunteered for the nursing staff. Both thought they could also save us some money by cleaning the office each evening. But after one day of working at the office and staying after hours to vacuum and mop floors, they told us in no uncertain terms to hire a cleaning woman. We also needed to employ a full-time nurse—ideally, a person older than ourselves to lend some maturity to our staff. We figured that someone from the area would be valuable in helping us know the community, so we hired a local, licensed practical nurse, a woman who appeared to be quiet and knowledgeable. We really didn't know how to interview a prospective employee and knew nothing about background checks or references.

Within a few days of hiring her, I was setting up a checking account and a line of credit at the State Bank of Markle when the president asked to see me. After some small talk about being glad to have us in Markle, he said, "You've made your first mistake. You've hired as your nurse someone who has emotional problems and whose gossiping has caused bad feelings in the community. Many folks won't come to your office if she is there."

Lee and I discussed this new difficulty and decided it was better to deal with it before we opened the doors. So we fired our first employee before we ever started. We told her we decided on a registered nurse rather than a licensed practical nurse to run our office. She accepted this gracefully and remained our friend and patient for the rest of her life.

Luckily, when it came to hiring staff, we had a quick learning curve. That first year we engaged Kathryn Thomas, a registered nurse with strong leadership skills. She eventually managed our staff and worked for us until she retired. We didn't know it at the time, but when we hired Kathryn, we were gaining the fix-it services of her husband, Floyd, a local farmer who could take care of anything broken, from machinery to tree limbs.

Mary was delighted when we hired Clara Cart to take turns with her at the reception desk. Fortunately for us, Clara also worked at the office until she retired. Soon Ruby Kreisher joined our staff as a custodian, but we never saw her much since she cleaned at night, when the office was empty. We hired Ruby's daughter, Linda Reed, in 1966, first as a receptionist and later as a bookkeeper and an office administrator. Linda's good judgment helped guide the medical center for forty-five years.

As part of setting up our office, we had to decide what to charge for an office call since among doctors the fees varied. The Gitlin brothers in Bluffton provided some assistance in that respect. Max, the oldest, started his practice before World War II. Both he and his brother, Bill, served in the war and then came back to Bluffton where they had grown up. They told us they charged four dollars for an office call and that included any medicine they gave. With that set fee, we figured it would take us years to show a profit. Then we found out they only charged for an office call if they prescribed medicine. However, every month when patients came for refills on their prescriptions, they paid four dollars even if they never saw a doctor.

Lee and I decided to charge four dollars for an office call, one dollar for a urinalysis, and a fee for medicine based on the cost of each drug. We would mostly carry generic medicines, and most of these we would bottle ourselves before dispensing.

As a child, I saw the doctor for all the common childhood diseases and to have my tonsils and adenoids removed, but, otherwise, I was seldom sick. I spent little time in the doctor's office on my own accord, but I remember going with my mother, Lucile, when she needed to see a physician. We traveled about ten miles to LaGrange to see Dr. Flannigan. He never gave appointments; we had to check into a crowded waiting room and wait our turn. Sometimes, after sitting for several hours, we would learn that the doctor was now at the hospital and might be in later or might not. Because of the time I spent squirming in a chair, looking at pictures in farm magazines, or sitting on the front steps watching cars and Amish buggies drive past, I always disliked going to Dr. Flannigan's office. Of course, it didn't help that after that long wait I might be rewarded for my patience with a shot in the bottom.

I didn't want this long waiting period for my patients, but the doctors in the area tried to dissuade us from scheduling appointments. Bill Gitlin said, "Appointments won't work. Patients don't expect to make an appointment, and, if you set up times but your patients don't show, you'll be sitting there with nothing to do until the next person with an appointment arrives. It just won't work." He also said that we'd need to offer evening hours since patients sometimes couldn't come during the day. Bill and Max alternated nights so that a doctor was in the office every weekday evening.

Lee and I talked it over and decided that we would have appointments like the younger doctors in the cities did. We also decided to keep the office open only one night a week—on Monday, from 7 to 9. Like Markle's bank and most of its stores, our office would close on Thursday afternoons and offer Saturday morning hours. Anticipating that we wouldn't be busy at first, we brought in a chessboard.

Our open house was on March 8th, but I saw my first patient two weeks earlier. Lee and I were papering a mural of a wooded lake to the waiting room wall when Richard Randol, a high school senior, walked in. He told us he needed a physical exam to apply for college. Richard entered a room of sawdust and molding and saw two men wearing nail aprons. He told me later that he wondered, "What kind of doctors are these?"

My next patient came in during our Sunday open house, a thirteen-year-old boy whose father rushed him past the welcoming line. This boy had been burning a fence row of weeds when his clothes caught fire. The nurse and I spent the rest of the open house cleaning, debriding, and dressing the first and second degree burns.

On Wednesday, March 11th, the Markle Medical Center officially opened. I was there alone since I had started my internship four months before Lee. I saw twenty patients. That was the slowest day we ever had in our office. The appointment book continued to fill up even when Lee joined me in July.

Since most Markle businesses closed on Thursday afternoons, Lee and I shut down our office, too, and spent our free afternoons golfing together. Or, rather, *trying* to golf together. So many urgent phone calls would summon us from the course we decided to break town tradition and keep the office open. We continued Monday evening hours for about two years, until we perfected our scheduling to the point we could see all of our patients during the daytime. We often didn't leave the office until 6 or 7 p.m., but then we didn't have to return that night—at least not for appointments.

We never used the chessboard.

THE BOYS

Lee and I came to Markle confident we were real doctors—with framed degrees to prove it. However, some of our patients weren't as convinced. They seemed to agree with the first part of Benjamin Franklin's advice: "Beware of the young doctor and the old barber." From the onset our office was busy, but we'd repeatedly hear, "You look too young to be a real doctor." Since I was six years Lee's junior, I'd hear this even more often than he.

We would tell these dubious patients what was wrong and then prescribe their cure. Maybe they needed surgery or hospitalization. They would listen patiently and then say, "I'll think about it, and let you know what I decide." Several days later we would discover they had been admitted to the local hospital in Bluffton or Huntington by another doctor for the same surgery or illness we had discussed.

You might wonder how we gained this intelligence. In the 1960s no local news was too minor for *The Bluffton News Banner* to report. In fact, readers fondly nicknamed it *The Bluffton Blabber*. They might find their traffic ticket listed on the front page or a description of who they had for company on Sunday. *The Banner* especially valued hospital news. Admissions and releases had their own column. Naïve about the paper's rigorous pursuit of hospital knowledge, I ran into the editor one day during morning rounds and had what I took to be a casual conversation about a patient's recovery. The next day my off-the-cuff remarks were the basis of a full-blown news story and the hospital administrator gave me clear instructions to never discuss patients with *The Banner.*

Lee and I grew tired of hearing ourselves called *The Boys*, a nickname that seemed to overemphasize our youth and inexperience. After some thought, we decided that one way to engender community confidence might be to let our hair grow. This was the 60s, but we both had flattops from our high school days. I didn't really want to get rid of mine. Though the fashion was now longer, I liked the ease of caring for such short hair. Some members of Forks Mennonite Church had seen my flattop as worldly, in the same league as class rings and bow ties, but my parents had been more progressive and never criticized my haircut. Several more inches of hair did make Lee and me appear older, and the additional time it took to groom was balanced by fewer trips to the barber.

So haircuts helped, but what really seemed to establish our credibility that first summer was an experience I had treating a young woman whose physical ailments were so mysterious they had been diagnosed as psychological. One evening this woman's husband called to ask if I would see his wife who was having trouble walking. It was not an emergency, but I told him to bring her to the office and I would see her. At that point, most people in the community were new to me and I hadn't met either the wife or her husband. As I waited at the front window, a car pulled to the curb and a man walked around to lift a petite woman out of the passenger seat. I opened the office door, and the man carried her back to an examination room.

The woman told me that she had been gradually losing strength in her legs. "I haven't had any kind of accident or injury," she explained. "A year ago I just started noticing that my legs were weaker. After the birth of our third daughter, that weakness got worse. For the last several months, I've needed a wheelchair. I can't even take care of my children. My parents care for me and the children while my husband is at work."

The husband then explained how they had visited many doctors and several specialists but no one had been able to diagnose his wife's problem. X-rays and tests showed nothing abnormal. One doctor recommended a psychiatrist.

I said I wanted to do a complete physical examination and then we would discuss the options.

Let me sidetrack to explain why I felt it was so important that I perform a thorough exam. It wasn't just because all through medical school my teachers at Indiana University had said, "The best way to understand a patient's illness is to listen carefully to his or her story and then perform a complete physical exam." It was also because when it came time to see my first patient, I failed to follow that advice.

In the fall of 1961 I was a third-year medical student just starting my clinical experience and feeling nervous about moving from books and cadavers to real patients. My first patient was in his early fifties and at four hundred pounds easily filled the width of his hospital bed. There were about forty other beds in the men's ward, so I pulled the curtain around us and then tried to start a conversation. But it was difficult. He mostly answered my questions with a *yes* or *no*, and when he did attempt to explain anything, he was hesitant, as if slow-witted. Flustered, I hurried through the interview. After all, he had been transferred to the IU Medical Center because of increased weakness and severe thirst, and it seemed pretty obvious to me that he was an undiagnosed diabetic with obesity and hypertension.

If taking the patient's history had been awkward, examining his body was more so. His corpulence made a physical exam difficult, as did the foul-smelling creases in his skin. Again, I rationalized that because I had my diagnosis a thorough exam wasn't really necessary.

Later that morning I met with Dr. John B. Hickam, the chair of medicine and a renowned educator and physician. I stood in a circle with him and several other interns to present my opinion as to my patient's illness and treatment.

"Gerald," he said, adjusting his horn-rimmed glasses and looking straight at me, "what did you think of this man's inability to urinate standing up?"

I said I thought it was from his obesity.

"Did you check his genitalia?"

I had to admit that I had not.

"Your patient doesn't have any external genitalia," said Dr. Hickam. "His testicles are small and withdrawn from a severe case of Klinefelter's Syndrome, a genetic condition that affects physical and cognitive development. The family doctor who saw him for many years never realized he had this condition either."

I wanted to shrink into my shoes. Because I had lacked the perseverance to ask enough questions and complete the exam, I hadn't gotten my patient's whole history—only a piece of it. He certainly was diabetic, but Klinefelter's explained his halting speech and some of his muscular weakness. Soon my embarrassment was coupled by guilt. Here was someone who had undoubtedly experienced a traumatic childhood and adolescence—taunted for his weakness and learning disabilities, forced to endure the humiliation of PE showers. Here was a person who with the aid of a caring, astute physician could have received hormone treatments that would have made his life easier. I started to see this man in a larger context and wished I had given him the gift of my time.

I promised myself that from then on I would honor my patients with the attentiveness and thoroughness I observed in Dr. Hickam. That's why now, after checking my patient's vital signs, I started a thorough test of her muscles, sensations, and reflexes.

When I performed a Babinski's Test on her left foot, she responded positively. Dr. Babinski, who lived in Paris from 1857-1931, is remembered for his discovery that when the big toe dorsiflexes (sticks straight up) upon stimulation of the sole, it's a sign of lesions in the pryramidal nerve tract, an indication that there is an organic lesion as distinguished from a hysteric hemiplegia (psychological paralysis). This one finding indicated that the patient had a real problem and not an imagined weakness. I told her that a lesion somewhere along the nerve paths to her lower legs was causing her problems and that we would take more x-rays of her back and compare them with previous ones.

When the new hospital x-rays came back, they revealed a destructive lesion in the seventh and eighth thoracic vertebras. Something was destroying the vertebra in her upper back. Checking previous records, I discovered that only lower back x-rays were ever ordered.

I sent the patient to a neurosurgeon I knew from my internship. Before surgery we thought the lesion might be cancerous, but it turned out to be a benign neurofibroma (nerve tumor) and was almost completely removed. Immediately, the woman began to gain strength in her legs. Soon walking wasn't her challenge, but readjusting to the role of caregiver to three young children—a much happier task and one she successfully tackled.

The story of the woman's remarkable recovery made the rounds, and patients who were once apprehensive showed more confidence—though to what extent that was due to the patient's recovery, our longer hair, or just getting to know us, I don't know.

TWO: THE FIRST YEARS

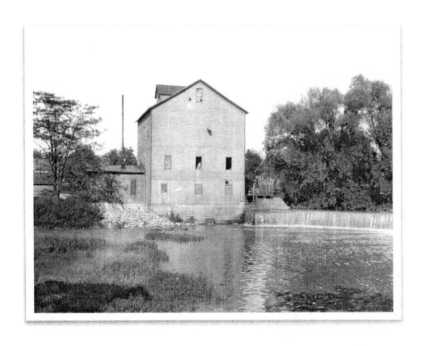

SETTLING IN

When Mary and I moved from Fort Wayne to Markle, her dad drove down and transported our possessions in his grain truck. We hadn't accumulated much—some secondhand furniture and a sixteen-inch black and white television. When Marlis' baby bed, which was once mine, fell apart during the move, one of the women who had come to welcome us, Helen Bates, went home and returned with her own child's outgrown crib.

That first year we rented a house at the northwestern outskirts of Markle, on Logan Street (State Route 224). This white, black-shuttered Cape Cod had been recently moved from land cleared to form the Huntington Reservoir. Our neighbors made us feel welcome, but it was difficult to keep their surnames straight with all the Bears, Foxes, Wolfs, and Beavers. Shari entered the house one afternoon saying she had just talked to a nice lady down the street. When Mary asked who the woman was, she replied, "Oh, one of those people with an animal name."

We moved during the first week of March expecting pleasant weather for the rest of the spring, but that same month a severe cold spell set in, with a snowstorm stranding cars and semi-trailers for thirty-six hours on the highway in front of our house. A young registered nurse we hired, Nancy Kunnert from Fort Wayne, was marooned and stayed at our house overnight. Nancy slept in Shari's bedroom, and before she turned off the light, Shari showed her a lost tooth she'd been hiding. "Don't tell my parents, but I lost this today," she said. "I'm going to put it under my pillow and see if there really is a tooth fairy." Nancy told us later that proving the tooth fairy's existence was one of the nicest things she ever got to do.

Nancy did many other kind things. She baked our daughters a coconut Easter cake in the shape of a bunny and treated patients at the office, especially the children, with compassion and respect. Unfortunately, Nancy was a Type 1 diabetic who had poor kidneys. After her second year with us, she moved back to her parents' home in LaPorte, Indiana where she started dialysis and died just a few years later.

Our first winters in Markle were extremely cold, but we soon discovered how townspeople and farmers coped with long stretches of freezing weather. They invited us to the river to skate on a half-mile area cleared of snow—just above the Markle Dam. We had to avoid areas along the river edge where springs weakened the ice, but those who had skated on the river for years knew those places well. On the bank, we'd light a campfire and perch on logs to warm our feet or toast marshmallows. After Lee and I finished at the office, we'd often meet our families and friends for a wiener roast with a pot of baked beans before an evening of skating. I was surprised at what skilled skaters and hockey players the townspeople and farmers were. They told us skating stories from the first half of the century and tales about tobogganing down Wolfcale's Hill on long sleds fashioned from the tin of a barn roof.

On summer nights, distant cheering drew the Millers and the Kinzers to the softball field on the south side of the river. My favorite fast-pitch softball teams to watch were Heller Stone and Kreischer Phillips 66. In mid-August, they played in the Markle Softball Tournament, a sixteen-team invitational event that boasted the best teams in

Northeastern and Central Indiana. This tourney took place over eight nights and drew over a thousand people to the bleachers or to watch from inside cars or on their hoods. Horns honked in a chorus for home runs. Cars parked so near to the field that sometimes a fly ball cracked a windshield, and once, when a ball pierced an auto's cloth top, the outfielder reached in to grab it. Markle often hosted the State Softball Tournament, as well; this competition lured teams from all over Indiana. Lee played first base for Kriescher with considerable skill. I wasn't much of an athlete, but later, as President of Lions Club, I did help organize the Lionesses, a women's softball team.

The town paid the electric bill for the lighted ball field, and Psi Iota Xi women ran the concession stand that sold hot dogs and breaded veal sandwiches. My daughters developed a taste for the concession stand beverages called "suicides"—mixtures of Mountain Dew, Sprite, A&W Root Beer, and Pepsi. The popular candy was red licorice—stiff hollow tubes chewed off at the ends to use as straws. When Marlis and Shari weren't rooting for the local farm, little league, and pony league baseball teams, they were at the playground, gripping the iron railing of the merry-go-round or standing in line for the slick, aluminum slide.

The park, owned by the Markle Fish and Game Club, was the pride of the town; its swimming pool, a former limestone quarry, attracted people from surrounding communities, including Fort Wayne. Eventually, the Fish and Game Club added two lighted tennis courts and offered summer lessons. I joined the doubles league since with doubles more finesse was required. . .and less running.

41

Summer or winter, my family's favorite place was a covered bridge two miles east of Markle. This double-span bridge was over two hundred feet long and completed in 1870 on land donated by a farmer named Cover. To reach Cover Bridge we drove or rode our bikes down a curving dirt road, a lover's lane overhung by boughs of old ash trees. In summer, we'd take picnics of barbecued chicken and cast our lines for rock bass and sun fish. Older people could remember when school girls in white frocks brought their easels to paint views of the bridge. They also recalled that when sunlight struck at just the right angle the past reappeared on the interior boards in the form of placards for Red Front Drug Store and Herron's Barber Shop. Everyone was saddened when arsonists in late May of 1966 destroyed Cover Bridge.

A year later the most interesting building in Markle—the Old Thomas Mill—also burned down and no one knew the culprits. Built in 1858, the mill was even older than the covered bridge. Both structures had been condemned by the state's Corp of Engineers as standing in the way of the new Wabash Reservoir Project.

During the last half of the 60s, the small-town community we were just beginning to know underwent a time of transition: schools were consolidated, the reservoir project was finished, a four-lane highway—I-69—was being built near its outskirts. All of these were large projects with ramifications for a small town like Markle.

ETA

Initially, Lee and I figured we'd be using two hospitals when we set up our practice: Lutheran, where we were interns, and Huntington, the hospital closest to Markle. But this plan changed when a group of four Fort Wayne anesthesiologists asked if we'd assume their responsibilities at the nearby Wells County Hospital. Traveling to Bluffton was inconvenient for them, and they were busy enough with work in Fort Wayne. Lee and I agreed, and so the last months of our internships were especially busy as these physicians trained us in anesthesiology.

When Bluffton physicians William and Max Gitlin learned that Lee and I could administer anesthesia, they also wanted us to give it to their patients needing surgery. So as our Markle practice began, I was not only admitting patients to Lutheran and Huntington Hospitals, but also driving to Wells County Hospital almost every morning and occasionally after office hours for emergencies. To make my schedule more complicated, each of these three hospitals was in a different direction from Markle: Lutheran was twenty miles to the north; Huntington, ten miles to the west; and Wells County, twelve miles to the east.

Years later to make long car rides more interesting, I'd play an ETA (Estimated Time of Arrival) guessing game with my youngest child, Steve, who was born in 1967. I was typically the winner, not only because my foot regulated the gas pedal, but also because I had a lot of experience gauging how long it would take me to reach my patients. Traveling between three hospitals not only developed my ETA skills early on but my ability to estimate other things, like the arrival of babies.

Early one Saturday afternoon, about two months after the office opened, my first OB patient went into labor. This young woman, who happened to be my next-door neighbor, had chosen to give birth to her first child at Huntington Hospital. I wanted everything to go perfectly. I checked her at the hospital and estimated that it would be a number of hours till she would deliver. I would have plenty of time to drive to Lutheran where that morning I had admitted a seventy-year-old man with a bleeding gastric ulcer. However, when I reached the fourth floor at Lutheran, a nurse told me that she had just received a call from Huntington Hospital saying they needed me immediately for a delivery. I dashed to my car and headed straight back to Huntington. Speeding through Roanoke on Highway 24, I heard a siren and in my rear-view mirror spied a state trooper's flashing light.

I pulled over and waited while the officer checked my license plate number. Then he slowly got out of his car and ambled up to my side window.

Leaning down, he drawled, "Do you know how fast you were going?"

I told him I didn't know, but I was in a hurry to get to Huntington Hospital to deliver a baby.

"Well, all right, then, go on ahead, but drive carefully," he said with measured words. "We need all of our doctors."

Fifteen minutes later, I arrived in the delivery room just in time to catch the baby, but the nurses were laughing. They said the policeman had called to make sure I had been telling the truth. I was still wearing my flattop then, and he might have had doubts that I was even old enough to be a physician.

Of course, after the baby was delivered I drove back to Lutheran again, to check on my elderly patient. That day I felt like I had literally met myself coming and going.

Over the next several months I delivered more babies at Huntington Hospital, but as more doctors asked me to give anesthesia at Wells County Hospital, the logistics of trying to serve three hospitals grew increasingly difficult. It was during this frenzied time that I adopted the habit of eating my breakfast—usually one or two bananas—on the road. "I have to look out on my way to work or I'll slip on your banana peels," one Wells County RN used to tell me, though I'm confident most peels landed safely in the ditch. Finally, I got wise (or just run down) and started asking my OB patients if it was okay with them if they delivered at Wells County Hospital. Without exception, they all said they would go wherever I preferred.

Patients appreciated the tender care of the Bluffton nurses and the hospital's family-like atmosphere. I liked the atmosphere, too. It was a place where everyone got along, and I could get to know people, no matter their job; I could sit down for a cup of coffee with the janitor or a slice of peach pie with the pharmacist. As an added bonus, the kitchen workers, all of whom were from the local community, were excellent cooks. In fact, their homemade dishes were so tasty that people treated the hospital cafeteria like a restaurant and ate there on Sundays.

After several years Lee and I weren't going to Huntington Hospital anymore, except for emergencies. We liked the staff there, but it was a relief to not be pulled in three directions. We still sent patients to Lutheran Hospital, but only when they needed specialized care that couldn't be provided at Bluffton. As the years passed, more specialists, such as cardiologists, urologists, and oncologists, came to Wells County Hospital for specialized clinics. Only once in forty-two years did we have to call an anesthetist from Lutheran, and that was for a high-risk patient who was also a nurse in our surgical unit. By 1969 so many patients from surrounding counties were coming to Wells County Hospital that the hospital board changed its name to Wells Community Hospital.

Over the years I grew adept at predicting my travel time to that hospital. But late one night in the early 90s, on my way to see a patient with trouble breathing, an unforeseen circumstance caused me to radically misjudge my ETA. That's because I ended up walking three of those 12.5 miles. I was still about five miles from the hospital when a flat tire pulled me to the roadside. To make matters worse, I had rushed from the house without bothering to put on a coat and gloves even though it was winter. Trying to change that tire was a cold, bitter task. My flashlight batteries were dead, and I couldn't figure out how to even unlock my new car's hubcap. I fumbled around for a while but soon gave up.

Traffic was scarce, and it was too dark to hitch-hike anyway. Now and then I'd come to a house, but no one would respond to the doorbell or my knocks.

At the edge of Bluffton I reached the pretzel factory where the nighttime shift let me in to phone the hospital for a ride. I arrived, greasy and half-frozen, but I cared for my patient and then slept in the doctors' lounge until time for morning rounds.

The thoughtful hospital maintenance staff changed my tire that night and a few days later Mary and Steve bought me my first cell phone.

Hoosier author Jessamyn West once observed, "A taste for irony has kept more hearts from breaking than a sense of humor, for it takes irony to appreciate the joke is on oneself." I think I have that taste for irony. I can appreciate that one of the reasons I wanted to practice medicine in a small town was to experience a leisurely lifestyle.

I can also appreciate that, though I became pretty good at predicting my time on the road and the arrival of babies, I never became proficient at judging my ETA for evening dinner. In fact, Mary says I was a miserable failure at that.

HOUSE CALLS

During our first years at Markle, Lee and I made numerous house calls—before, during, and after office hours, some scheduled, some not. It was still a common practice then for physicians in rural areas to make home visits to see infants and to treat children with infectious diseases such as chicken pox and measles. In a few years, though, as their confidence in us grew, parents started bringing their children to the office, realizing that they could be seen more quickly and without added risk.

I soon discovered another reason for so many house calls: ill patients insisted on staying at home as long as possible before being admitted to the hospital. At first I figured this hesitancy was due to the cost of hospital care. But room rates were quite reasonable at that time—sixteen dollars per day—and a hospital nurse told me it wasn't due to that concern.

"People see that patients in hospitals are dying," she explained, "so they think you're hospitalized because you are going to die. They wait until they cannot possibly live any longer at home, and, sure enough, they go to the hospital and die."

Lee and I knew we had to change this mindset. We tried to create a positive view of what a hospital was—a place to recover and go home.

Another reason for so many house calls was because our hospital in Bluffton didn't have an emergency room yet. Instead of telling patients I'd meet them at the hospital, I either drove to their homes or opened up the office.

Sometimes, of course, I made a house call as an immediate response to an emergency. There was no 911 at that time and no ambulance service with a medical team— only the funeral director who transported patients in a converted hearse. One rainy Saturday afternoon a farm wife called, saying, "My husband is back in the field, lying up against the fence and holding his chest." I knew she lived about three miles from Markle, so I told her I'd be there in a few minutes and to call the funeral home for the ambulance.

When I arrived, I grabbed my medical bag and portable oxygen tank and jogged to the back of the farmer's sheep field. It had started to rain hard, and spears of lightning angled straight down. I was worried that the farmer might get struck, so the first thing I did was pull him away from the wire fencing. He was pale and sweaty and said he felt a crushing pain in his chest. I gave him an injection of morphine and started him on oxygen while we waited for the ambulance. This was before angioplasty, stents, and coronary by-passes, but the farmer, who was in his mid-fifties, survived and went on to live fifteen more years.

One day an urgent call came while I was seeing a patient at the office: "I just found my mother—she's blue and isn't breathing!" Our head nurse, Kathryn, rattled off quick instructions on how to find the house as I was heading out the door. I sped north for two miles and ran to the house and into a bedroom where an elderly woman lay motionless on a bed. She was blue but still warm, with a weak, thready pulse. There was no breathing. I pulled up on her chin to open her airway—and still, no breath. Then I ran my fingers through her mouth and felt something solid at the tip of my index finger. Reaching into her throat with two fingers, I pulled out

49

a thick hunk of roast beef—two inches long and an inch wide. The woman gasped. Soon, she was pink and alert.

Another afternoon while seeing a patient I was interrupted with the alarming news that an older married couple had been found unconscious in their living room. A neighbor who knew they were home but received no answer when she knocked had discovered them. I rushed to their Markle address and ascertained both were still breathing. I also heard the faint rumble of an engine—from what sounded like the basement.

A few houses in Markle are built into the hill slope that faces the river. These homes sometimes have garages directly below the main level. You drive in under your house where your car stays warm in the winter and cool in the summer. You can take a stairway right up to your living quarters. This set-up is great unless you forget to turn off the car engine.

When I heard that motor running, I flung open the doors and windows and raced downstairs to switch off the ignition. Even before the ambulance had arrived, my patients regained their consciousness, recovering from a heavy dosage of carbon monoxide.

Sometimes emergency calls were due to a patient's adverse reactions to a medication. One Thanksgiving evening I was called to a home in Markle where one of the guests, a middle-aged patient of mine, had developed stiffness in his one hand. I say "one hand" because his other had been lost in a corn-picker accident. The remaining hand was now drawing back and my patient could feel his back arching. He was also having difficulty chewing and swallowing.

When I asked if he was taking any medication, the family showed me a bottle of Compazine tablets. This drug treated acute nausea and vomiting, and I carried it in my medical bag, in many variable dosages. Available as pills, suppositories, or injectables, Compazine was rapidly effective, making it an ideal drug. The family said my patient's orthopedic surgeon had sent the pills home with him in case he had nausea. Because my patient wanted to make sure he enjoyed his large Thanksgiving meal, he had been taking the drug regularly all day, but he hadn't attributed his increasing stiffness to the drug since he was taking it as directed.

During my pediatric clerkship at Riley Hospital, I had seen a preteen brought in by ambulance who exhibited similar symptoms to this man's. The boy was having an adverse reaction to Compazine, and the emergency doctor treated him with Benadryl. Fortunately, I carried that drug in my medical bag. So there in the living room I gave my patient an injection. Within minutes his arms, legs, and back relaxed. He started talking and was soon laughing at himself.

During the next several months, Lee and I handled a few more incidents related to Compazine reactions. I called the orthopedic group from Fort Wayne to explain what was happening and suggest that when they discharged their patients they give them three tablets to take home instead of twenty. That simple measure took care of the Compazine problem.

Seeing a patient in his or her home meant I could sometimes get a better notion for the source of a mysterious illness. One spring I received a call from a fifty-year-old woman who lived with her aged parents. She was having persistent vomiting and felt too dizzy to drive to the office. My examination revealed that her symptoms were more generalized than just the stomach flu and not triggered by an inner-ear problem. They started suddenly with no apparent cause. I gave her an injection for the vomiting and several suppositories. She soon recovered but her illness remained a mystery—until the next house call.

The following spring, I received another call from her. She had the same symptoms, only worse. I again drove to the farm. I knew if she previously had the stomach flu it wasn't likely she had it again. I quizzed her about her diet and asked whether she ate anything that her parents did not eat. She said, "No, I haven't eaten anything out of the ordinary."

But then her father who was sitting in the same room spoke up: "Yes, you have. You ate those puffball mushrooms from the pasture." He went on to tell me that he and his wife wouldn't eat them as they weren't morel mushrooms.

"I thought they had to be okay since they tasted so good," my patient said.

If I hadn't gotten a clue from her father, I might never have figured out that this woman was poisoning herself.

Since I had no cell phone, GPS, or even a scout's compass to point my direction, the most difficult part of a house call could be reaching my patient, especially at night and when the call came from unfamiliar territory, sometimes quite distant. My most remote destination for a house call was to a residence on the western edge of Huntington County. It took me an hour to reach this patient, and when she eventually became an invalid, I made that journey a number of times. Navigation to patients was made easier by the fact that Indiana townships and counties are mostly square and that country roads, unless they're near a river, usually intersect at right angles about every mile. Permanent landmarks such as churches, schools, and graveyards proved useful, and early on I learned the names of very small towns that were almost ghost towns, towns where my touchstone might be a Mom-and Pop grocery store, grain elevator, mechanic's garage, or just a few houses or old, empty buildings.

Sometimes the difficulty in reaching patients was due to insufficient directions. Lee received a call late one night from an aged man who said his wife was sick and couldn't breathe. "I'll keep a light on," the man said and then abruptly hung up without giving his name or address. Lee didn't know what to do but to open our office and call the emergency rooms of the three nearest hospitals to see if anyone was waiting for him. He kept hearing the man's voice repeat, "I'll keep a light on." Lee finally decided to just look until he found a house with a light on. He chose a direction at random and drove. Soon he saw a light—it was the right home. The woman was seriously ill, and Lee sent her straight to the hospital.

On a winter night when large drifts banked the roads, another elderly gentleman called to tell me his wife had a high fever and a cough. They lived along the Wabash River, west of Markle and back a long lane. He told me the snow was deep in the lane—I would need to park by the highway and travel by foot. When I arrived, the electricity was out and there were no porch lights or house lights to guide me down the lane. With no illumination except from the moon, I knew I'd have trouble finding my patient, so I stumbled to a nearby house to borrow a flashlight. Then I cut through a field to reach the patient's home.

She was lying on the floor, near the warmth of a fireplace. The only other light emanated from the low gleam of a lantern and a few candles. I examined her and after making a diagnosis of pneumonia, gave her an injection and a supply of antibiotics and mucolytics. Though the contents of my medical bag were modern, that night I felt as if I had traveled through the snowdrifts of the past to reach a little house on the prairie.

I felt more up-to-date during the blizzard of 1978 when highways and roads through Markle drifted shut and I zipped to house calls on the back of a snowmobile. The fleet that formed to aid stranded motorists also helped me reach my patients.

My family lived two miles from town by then, too far for me to make it home from the office. Fortunately, Bruce and Linda Meyers, the local mortician and his wife, put me up. But I didn't see them much. That first evening I was surprised to discover how many people don't realize they are running out of medicine until the bottle is empty. We had our new office by then, one with an independent pharmacy attached, and people either walked over or rode on snowmobiles to fetch their medicines. I spent much of the evening at the counter, preparing prescriptions for patients who were out of insulin, heart, or blood pressure medicine. I left notes for the pharmacist so he knew what to charge the next time they came in.

Some house calls could be pleasant and relaxing—accompanied by a cup of coffee or a glass of iced tea. I especially enjoyed visiting the storytellers, people like Mr.

Rittenhouse, who was a hundred years old and lived with his daughter and her husband on Union Center Road. He was bedfast but maintained a cheerful disposition. My daughter, Marlis, liked to go along, and I assumed that was because she enjoyed hearing him rib me about charging ten dollars just to change his catheter or because he told us stories about his younger days. But she says now that what drew her was the jar of hard candy Mr. Rittenhouse always offered. One of his stories I still remember is about the time he decided to start courting and needed his first suit. Since one of his friends was of courting age, too, they went shopping together in Markle. Each bought a spiffy suit for four dollars, took it home, and then decided they didn't like it so much, after all. But since they remembered liking each other's new suit, they happily enacted an exchange.

Occasionally, I'd be called on a house call that wasn't necessary. Once, a patient phoned during office hours, asking me to stop by his house on my way home. When I arrived, I discovered he had been at work all day and only had a head cold. I asked why he hadn't come to the office for an appointment, and he said, "Your charge for a house call is so low that it works better for me to have you come to my house and see me. I don't have to wait in your office or miss any work."

After that, I asked the nurse to obtain more information before scheduling a house call and we also increased the difference between the cost of an office and a home visit.

One night at about two in the morning, I received a call from a patient who was a school teacher. She said she needed an injection to fall asleep. She just had to get to sleep. I didn't carry any sedatives in my medical bag so I met her at the office and gave her a shot. But then, when I arrived home, I couldn't fall asleep. As I lay waiting to get up again for morning rounds, I decided to never again make a night call for insomnia.

Our family had an unlisted phone number, but it wasn't long until many patients knew it. Some called me when I wasn't on call but usually just to give a progress report or ask a question. These calls bothered Mary more than they bothered me. When she gave our phone number to friends and acquaintances, she'd say, "This is my phone number—not Gerald's."

One elderly woman habitually called our home number early in the morning to ask me to see her ailing husband before I made my hospital rounds. She tried to phone early enough so that she could catch me before I left the house. But since I might leave anytime between 5 and 6 a.m., depending on how many patients I had to see, she sometimes called after I had left. In that case, Mary would have to get up to go around the bed to answer and then she couldn't get back to sleep. When this caller missed me, she'd call even earlier the next time. Sometimes it felt like we were all playing a game of tag, but this woman was such a nice person and clearly cared so deeply about her husband that I could never ask her to stop calling our home number. Eventually, the early morning house calls that started when her husband was in his eighties came to an end when he died in his nineties.

I can attribute the early morning hour of one house call to a train whistle. First, you should understand that until 1979 trains were an important part of Markle's history and culture. The Chicago & Erie line was completed in 1878, and two years later the town had doubled in size. Through the years, Markle people worked for the railroad, started new businesses related to the railroad, and played by the tracks when they were young. Doc Woods even attributed the high birthrate of Markle's "Incubator Avenue" to the 2:30 a.m. passenger train that roared through town.

By the time I arrived in Markle, the passenger train was no longer running, but there were still lots of freight trains that rumbled through, enough so that folks living close to the tracks organized their daily routine according to the whistles. The extent of this became clearer to me one morning after an elderly farmer called a little before 4:30, asking if I could check his wife who was feeling dizzy.

As the husband and wife spoke to me from their matching lazy-boys, I noticed that both were dressed for the day and seemed quite alert for such an early hour.

When I opened my medical bag to withdraw the blood pressure cuff, the husband said, "We wanted to catch you before you went on your hospital rounds." I said I was an early riser, but that I usually didn't go on my rounds as early as 4:30. The couple looked at each other in bewilderment and then at the wall clock.

"Oh, dear, we must have gotten up with the three o'clock train, instead of the five o'clock one," the wife said.

"I've already finished my chores," said her husband. "Now what do I do?"

When we moved to Markle, we had local telephone operators and party lines. I quickly learned that I should never say anything on the phone that I would not want public knowledge. But I did appreciate those operators. They almost always knew when I was making a house call in their area. While I was at one house, the phone might ring and it would be either the operator or a patient asking me to make another stop on my way home. This saved me from driving home and then going right out again. After several years our phone system changed to an efficient automatic system, but I missed that helpful network of operators.

Over the years the number of house calls I made decreased until I was only making from two to five a week. These visits were for elderly patients or those with chronic diseases such as cancer. It was rewarding to know that my visits could help someone avoid an emergency room visit, a hospital stay, or a move to the nursing home.

I always arranged a time for these house calls, but an older doctor in the area, who had practiced in Uniondale and Liberty Center, Dr. Gingerick, told me that he seldom scheduled his visits to the elderly or chronically ill—he just showed up. If he came at night while families were asleep, he wouldn't bother the household by knocking but just walk right in to see his patient since rural houses were seldom locked. Afterwards, he would leave a note for the family, along with medicine or maybe a prescription. I admired that level of trust between patients and families and doctors, but I was from a younger generation of doctors—a generation not so informal.

I scheduled my calls after hours or on Saturday mornings, times when I didn't have to be hurried and could converse with patients and their families about things other than just the patient's health. I had time to talk about sports or look at old photographs, a woodworking hobby, or maybe a collection of antique farm equipment. Such house calls might last an hour.

Or sometimes less. Once I walked into a farmhouse and was almost knocked back out by a strong, pervading odor like none I had ever encountered or imagined. I am sure the family found that smell pleasant. They welcomed me into a steamy kitchen where something was bubbling in kettles and congealing inside of glass jars. Pig brains. There were dozens lined up on the counters. I had eaten chocolate-covered caterpillars and kangaroo-tail soup, but imagining the flavor of those brains caused my stomach to turn over.

Before they could offer me a jar to take home, I had asked my patient the basic questions, pumped up the blood pressure cuff, and released the tension. I don't know the longest house call I ever made on a Saturday morning—but that was the shortest.

NIGHT DELIVERIES

It didn't take me long to discover that when the phone rang at night I could get more rest if I got out of bed and started the car. Otherwise, I'd lie awake wondering if the parent or spouse's appraisal was accurate.

Early one morning a worried mother called while it was still dark. Her seventeen-year-old daughter had awakened with severe abdominal pain. "This is unusual," she said. "She's just never sick."

As I drove to the office I considered possible reasons for the young woman's pain. It would be rare for appendicitis to come on this suddenly, but I had seen it happen. Or the pain could be from a ruptured ovarian cyst or a twisted ovary. Those problems could occur in a young woman, though this one seemed a little too young.

As I stood at the office door watching the patient get out of the car and walk towards me, I thought I had my diagnosis. I told her to lie down on an examining table, and then I felt her stomach. "Do you know that you're pregnant?" I asked. She smiled. I told her I was going to perform a vaginal examination since I was sure she was having labor pains. When I spread her legs, the baby's head was already crowning. With one push, the young mother gave birth to a seven-pound baby girl. The new grandmother was truly amazed. She had no idea her daughter was expecting, though she had noticed some recent weight gain.

Later that morning Janice Jordan, our nurse, was also more than mildly surprised when she opened the door to the examining room and discovered what I had been too exhausted to clean up. "What in the world happened in here?" she asked me.

Fortunately, most of my deliveries were in the hospital, though not always in the delivery room. Once I delivered a baby in the elevator and once in the public restroom. I was working as the emergency room physician when a woman dashed past me. I heard a scream from the bathroom and hurried inside just in time to lift a healthy six-pound baby boy from the commode. This gave new meaning to the term *a water-bath delivery.* "I wasn't having any pain," the first-time mother told me. "I just felt a pressure down below. When water started running down my leg, I thought I needed the bathroom."

I didn't mind getting up during the night for a hospital delivery because that was easier than having to leave a busy office during the day. After the twenty minute drive, there was the waiting period, the actual delivery, and then the drive back. When everything went smoothly, I was still away from the office for more than an hour and that would throw me way behind in seeing patients. Sometimes I could be away for two to three hours or more. The office nurses hated to see a daytime delivery because that meant rescheduling patients and dealing with complaints from those who waited.

But being alone in the delivery room at night with just one nurse and a nurse's aide could be stressful when there were complications. Being trained in multiple areas of medicine was helpful to me during those early years when there was little expertise at the hospital. I was called a General Practitioner then, and the title wasn't changed to Family Physician until I was in practice for about ten years.

My state license read "Physician and Surgeon," and this training in surgery and anesthesia was immensely useful when I needed to handle difficult births.

One night I had just delivered a spinal anesthetic to a woman in labor who was nearly ready to deliver. Most mothers, like this one, wanted to be awake to see their babies born, and I preferred that, too. As the spinal took hold, the patient's pain began to decrease and her legs grew numb. But then all of a sudden she had difficulty breathing and the numbness started spreading to her chest. I realized the anesthetic was reaching too high into her spinal column and that soon she would be paralyzed and unable to breathe.

I ordered the nurse to bring me the anesthetic machine from the major surgery room. Almost every morning I gave anesthetics for other doctors' surgery patients and so was familiar with supporting airways in order to keep patients alive. This time I also wanted to be sure I kept the unborn baby fully oxygenated. The expectant mother, who I had seen in prenatal visits, seemed relaxed and calm—not at all fearful. I supported her respirations for about ninety minutes until the spinal worked its way down and she was able to breathe on her own. I then went ahead and delivered a strong baby girl with a perfect Apgar score of ten.

Another night I was called to the hospital for the birth of a premature baby. The seventeen-year-old mother was the daughter of the nurse's aide assisting us that night in the delivery room. The young woman's water had broken, and she felt pressure with regular contractions. By the time I arrived, her baby, three months premature, was ready to be delivered. The delivery went well; the infant had good lungs and was active. But she was extremely small—one pound and fifteen ounces. In 1965 we had no neonatal intensive care or ambulance service to safely transport the infant to a referral hospital, no pediatrician at the hospital, and no visiting neonatologist who could travel to us in the middle of the night. So we started caring for this infant just as we would for all full-term babies—with some variations. We kept a nurse with her at all times, and she stayed in an incubator with controlled heat and oxygen. Because of her undeveloped central nervous system, she would often stop breathing. Then the nurse would stimulate the baby to take a breath by snapping against her feet.

The next morning we placed the infant on a rocking bed in the incubation unit. When this bed reached the bottom of a rotation, it jerked to start back up and this would stimulate the baby's breathing if it had stopped. We started feeding the infant small amounts of breast milk through a tiny catheter placed down the esophagus and into her stomach.

Eighteen years later, the mother of this baby brought her daughter to the office to meet me. They had both moved from the Markle area years before when the daughter was only a year or two old. That miracle baby who survived the odds was now a young woman eager for college.

I call her a "miracle baby," but every infant I delivered was a miracle. Each one reawakened my sense of wonder, reminding me that each breath I take--or anyone takes—is a manifestation of grace. C.S. Lewis could have been speaking of newborns when he wrote, "Miracles are a retelling in small letters of the very same story which is written across the whole world in letters too large for some of us to see."

THE DRAFT

In the autumn of 1965 the war in Southeast Asia was escalating. In April President Lyndon Johnson had deployed the first sixty thousand troops to Vietnam, and during the summer General Westmoreland launched the first major offensives against the Viet Cong. As United States' involvement intensified, the Selective Service began drafting doctors. Indiana needed to meet a quota of thirty-eight physicians between the ages of twenty-six and thirty-five. Lee was thirty-three, and I was twenty-seven. That fall we filled out our forms and went for our physicals in Indianapolis.

Our possible draft into the Vietnam War became a topic of concern in Markle. Soon a grassroots effort sprang up to obtain our exemption from service. The lead for an October 28th article in the *Community News* read: "What can a small town do when faced with the possible loss of doctors upon whom the health and welfare of the community depends? The answer can be found in Markle where residents are staging a community-wide effort to keep their clinic and the doctors who serve it." A citizens committee collected letters and circulated a petition addressed to the Selective Service and our political representatives. The petition recognized that doctors are needed in a military crisis but contended that they are also needed in small towns and rural communities. It mentioned that the community had recently labored to obtain their current doctors and were working vigorously now to keep them. In three days, the committee collected three thousand signatures. It even sent a letter to

President Johnson who promptly replied that "all possible consideration will be given."

U.S. Representative J. Edward Roush of Huntington came to town to meet with the committee. Six years earlier in 1959 the Congressman had gained the gratitude of Markle when he worked to save the town park from destruction. The reservoir project, an undertaking intended to control flooding hundreds of miles away in the southern reaches of the Wabash, was then in its planning stage, and the Army Corps of Engineers had determined the pool, the softball field, and the Boy Scout cabin would all be part of the reservoir. Fortunately for Markle, Congressman Roush convinced the Corps to save the fifty-acre park by building the levee around it. Now, as he heard the committee's concerns and asked questions, he struck me as a good listener and someone with a sincere interest in the welfare of small communities. He wasn't sure he could help our situation, but he said that if we were drafted, he would try.

Nine years earlier, when I was eighteen, I registered as a conscientious objector to war. My pacifist stance was formed by having grown up in the Mennonite Church where I was taught that Jesus' teachings are against the bearing of arms and that as one of his followers I'm called to treat even enemies with compassion. I recognized that there could be a serious cost to this path of nonviolence: Jesus ultimately died as a pacifist, and many sixteenth-century Mennonites were martyred for their refusal to take arms. During the French and Indian War, some of my ancestors were massacred when they wouldn't use their hunting rifles against a small band of Delaware renegades. During WWI, when conscientious objector status was not an option, a man from my home congregation was imprisoned for not answering the draft. I respected the men and women who did join the military, but my personal beliefs would not allow me to support the war effort, even as a physician.

When Indiana University School of Medicine mandated that I have a student deferment rank in order to be enrolled, I lost my conscientious objector status. Now I filed again as a CO which wasn't difficult since I was still a member of a historic peace church, though instead of Mennonite, it was Church of the Brethren. Mary and I contacted the central service agency of the Mennonite Church and discovered it had an opening for a doctor at its hospital in Puerto Rico, a site Selective Service approved for alternative service. If I was drafted, we decided we'd ask to serve there.

While we waited for our Selective Service letters, Lee and I hoped that only one of us would be drafted. That way the community would still have a doctor—though he might be chronically sleep-deprived.

When the letters arrived three months later, we discovered to our surprise that neither of us had been drafted. Lee's letter indicated he had passed his physical but was ineligible for the draft since he was over the age limit. My letter read that I had also passed the physical but was disqualified since I had begun my medical practice before March 1, 1964. The Selective Service was not drafting any doctor who was in practice as of that date.

Did someone along the paper trail fudge a few dates or definitions to keep us in Markle? We were too busy to ask.

ON MORSE STREET

For the first ten years of our practice, Lee and I worked in Dr. Woods' renovated office on Morse Street. This downtown location was especially nice during our office lunch breaks. Lee and I could walk over to the A & W drive-in to have a chilidog and root beer or to the corner drugstore's soda fountain for a sandwich and milkshake. Our favorite lunch spot, though, was the M & M Café.

Marjorie Souers and Mary Will whipped up delicious homemade pies and other menu items from the fruits and vegetables that Milward "Pop" Overholt supplied from his garden. Prices were reasonable: for only thirty-five cents, I could buy a hamburger, and for a dime, I could purchase a fresh sweet roll delivered from Heyerly's Bakery in Ossian. While at the café, Lee and I often conversed with other regulars, like the town's volunteer firemen, but we tried to time our meals so as to miss the daily influx of Madison Silo workers that slowed down the service.

Over lunch break I sometimes walked over to Randol's Barbershop for a haircut. Either Bill Randol or Ron Allred trimmed my hair. It didn't matter which; both were good barbers. But Bill was the storyteller. He knew a lot about the town's history, and some of his stories had been handed down to him from his father, Wade, who had also been a barber. In fact, the barbershop was a storehouse of information, not just concerning town history, but also current events. Old men and farmers and storekeepers with a day off—anyone who might in times past have sat around a store's pot-bellied stove—gathered in the warmth of Bill's barbershop to joke and share stories. While my hair was cut,

I could catch up on current events and hear commentary on crops and weather, fishing and politics. Mary could hear another version of local events when she went to get her hair done each week at Ramone's Beauty Salon.

Though Randol's Barbershop and Ramone's Beauty Salon were always busy, by the 60s Markle's downtown wasn't as thriving as it once had been. In the 20s and 30s shoppers could choose from four or five grocery stores. Now there was only one small grocery. From Bill and my older patients, I learned there was once a custom butchering shop, several dry goods stores, a men's clothing store, blacksmith and leather-working shops, a tire shop, shoe store, several fine restaurants, a Ford dealership, a movie theater, a prosperous hotel, and even a public gym that served as a roller rink and hosted an independent basketball tournament and operettas.

Better roads and discount chains now lured customers to Huntington, Bluffton, and Fort Wayne. Still, there were enough stores that, with the exception of buying clothes and groceries, Mary and I could do most of our shopping downtown. Businesses along Morse Street included Greenawalt's Furniture, Reed's Television, Hoover-Randol Hardware, Dr. Poppy's veterinarian office, Bott's Jewelry, Rainbow Tavern, Ramone's Beauty Salon, Markle Meat Freezer, M & M Café, a chair caning business, a dry clean delivery service, a couple of antique stores, and a corner drugstore. Around the corner on Clark Street was Hill's Market, Randol's Barber Shop, Pip Heron's Barber Shop, the A& W, and a gas station. We bought our first color television downtown, as well as a new dining room and living room set. Mary shopped for fresh fruit, vegetables, and meat from

Hill's Market, and I bought her an anniversary present at Bott's Jewelry. We purchased all of our insurance from my barber—Bill Randol.

It's hard for businesses in small towns to match the prices and selection of chains in the cities, but what small businesses in Markle had going for them was a tradition of integrity. I learned that this integrity might be remembered long after the owners died. I never had the pleasure of meeting Al Stauffer—he passed away in the 1954 Markle Memorial Day Parade with his tuba beside him—but I've been told what a good person he was and the slogan on his pencils: "Al Stauffer's Clothing—You Know Me."

When a business owner knows customers as more than customers—when they live next door or play in the same softball league or go to the same church—there's an added incentive to treat them fairly. In a town as small as Markle, if a business along Morse or Clark Streets didn't do sound work and treat its customers well, it couldn't stay in business for long. Word got around.

I noted this fairness when I bought my first office car—a 1965 Chevette—from Floyd "Red" Anderson at his dealership on Logan Street. I had some issues with that new car. I never complained to Red, but after he towed it a few times, he took the initiative to offer me a different vehicle. He did that out of courtesy and not because he legally had to. The Lemon Law (Motor Vehicle Protection Act) wasn't enacted by the Indiana Legislature until 1988.

Over the years, Mary and I never stressed much when we had problems with our cars because we knew we could trust the owners and mechanics at the Clark Street Markle 66 Garage, Marvin and Tom Highlen, to do excellent work at a reasonable price. There's less anxiety when your mechanic knows your car's history; less worry when your barber already knows how you want your hair cut; little or no stress when you trust your insurance agent to give you the best deal. In general, it's more relaxing to live in a place where you feel connected to the people you see and do business with. And, as more and more research is revealing, less stress means better health.

Since Markle is a river-town, in addition to being able to walk to other businesses from our office, I could also walk a few hundred feet and reach the Wabash. The name "Wabash" derives from *Ouabache,* the French spelling of the Algonquin word *Wah-Bah-Shik-Ki,* meaning "pure white," "water over white stones," or "it shines white." This name alludes to the fact that the river bottom in Huntington County is limestone and that the water was once transparent.

Of course, by the twentieth-century, run-off from farmland and industry insured that the water was no longer so clear. Still, the river was attractive. The scene toward the east was especially nice, offering a view of the Old Thomas Mill. This three-story structure was more than a hundred years old and for more than seventy years had been operated by four generations of the Thomas family: Enoch, Ansel, Claude, and Claude's sons, Ralph and Harold. The year we came to town, the mill's wood floor was still slick and polished. Its turbines produced flour that was sold in local grocery stores and had the reputation for the "best-ever" pie dough.

There's something romantic about a river-town, a place where you can cast a fish line from your back porch or ice skate behind Main Street. In 1930 Huntington historian Frank

S. Bash wrote in the *Huntington-Herald*: "Somehow, there has always been something inviting to an outsider in the town of Markle. Its people, its well-kept homes, picturesque river; mill-dam, bridge, general atmosphere and worthwhile history, made a strong and singular appeal to me." You feel near to nature as you eat bread made of wheat the river's power has ground. You sense life's mystery as you pause on a bridge, watching water flecked with sunlight flow toward the next bend.

One day, however, I had a view from the bridge that wasn't scenic or romantic. One morning, during our first or second year, Lee and I heard that something was happening at the river we had to see. During our lunch hour, we hurried to the bridge where a crowd was peering down at the river — or, rather, where the river used to be. Recently, the U.S. Army Corp of Engineers had diverted the Wabash for the reservoir project, so now the original river route through Markle was an oxbow, cut off from the river's new man-made channel by a levee with a control gate.

In the shallow water, thousands of desperate fish — most of them carp — were at the surface, flapping and gasping for air. People were in the water, too — lots of people — mostly men and women from Muncie who lived in a fishing camp of trailers and small cottages on the south bank, east of the bridge. These fishermen were wading toward three and four-foot fish and stabbing them with pitchforks!

Earlier that day the Department of Natural Resources had added a natural compound called Rotenone to the water. This chemical enters directly through the gills and inhibits cellular respiration, thus asphyxiating the fish. I don't remember why the fish were being killed — probably to control the carp population since carp are especially sensitive to that chemical. It was fascinating to see firsthand what leviathans lived in our local waters—but sad, too, since those fish fought for a breath they never could take.

When the Old Thomas Mill was condemned as standing in the way of the Wabash Reservoir Project, Mary and I hoped—along with many townspeople—that it might still be preserved as a historical museum or maybe a restaurant. But then one sad Sunday in 1967 the fire-whistle blew and we saw a column of leaping flames. The destruction of the mill was assigned to teenage vandals, but, as with the burning of the covered bridge one year earlier, no one was ever charged with the crime. Since the bridge had also been condemned by the Corp of Engineers, many people suspected that both events were somehow tied to the reservoir's construction.

Our downtown lost some of its charm with the destruction of the mill and the rechanneling of the river. But it was still a good place to run into friends, hear local news, and eat a tasty lunch. After the M & M closed, Billie Kreisher, opened a café at the same location. Lee and I also enjoyed our lunch breaks at this establishment, and forty-five years later I still savor the memory of Billie's homemade mince-meat pies.

THE QUARRY

On humid summer days, the Markle Pool drew lots of kids, including the Miller and Kinzer children who pedaled there on bikes. They could almost coast since the pool was at the bottom of Clark Street, just across the river.

In the 1920s the excavation of limestone from the Markle quarry ceased and the cavity was allowed to fill with clear, spring-fed water. This was a relief for storekeepers and nearby residents—dynamiting at the quarry shook buildings and broke windows. Once the digging stopped, the owners of the property, Joe and Goldy Cargar, permitted townsfolk to swim free of charge, as long as they were willing to share the shoreline with their dairy cows. A railroad line still lay at the bottom of the quarry as did a small building that once stored dynamite. It was a popular activity to dive down to the building's empty window, glide through, and then rocket back to the surface.

Even in the late 40s there were no lifeguards and no set hours. Families often came after supper to cool off. One of our Markle friends, Linda Pope, says her first childhood memory is swimming there on a summer night with her father: "I remember feeling it was just Dad and me under the stars with the occasional glow of swimmers' cigarettes in the dark while Mom watched with friends on the bank. Their gentle voices were muffled by the quiet splashes."

In 1950 the Markle Fish & Game Club under the leadership of Fay Geiger bought the quarry to preserve it as a public swimming area. They fenced in the five acres of water, hauled in fine sand for the beach, and added two water slides, diving boards, and a large and small raft. They built a cement building with showers and lockers and a concession area where children bought hot dogs, banana taffy, frozen Snickers, and snow cones. In the morning, before the pool opened, teachers offered swimming and water ballet lessons. Each summer at the annual Water Ballet, students performed synchronized swimming, along with a diving display and sometimes a dance on the sand with parasols or a hula dance. In the early 60s, they sang about surfing and a certain yellow polka-dot-bikini. The Markle churches held an annual "Galilean" service at the pool, with the minister preaching from a rowboat and the choir singing on the bank. The Markle Pool had more to offer than the usual small-town community pool; in fact, its sandy beach and spring-fed water drew families from as far away as Fort Wayne and Marion. Sometimes the pool was so packed on weekends that it had to shut its gates.

Our children learned to swim at the quarry. Marlis loved spending summer afternoons back flipping off the raft and diving from the rock ledges on the pool's undeveloped side. Steve, who worked several years as a lifeguard, would dive down to touch the railroad tracks, the wood ties lying by that time in haphazard positions. Snakes, mostly harmless ones, lived in the tall grass behind the pool, and one morning when he showed up for work, Steve had to help chase off a serpent sunning on the concrete near the concession stand.

The afternoon air smelled of Coppertone and the sand burnt bare feet. Blue gills nibbled toes. Teenagers liked to slip under the raft to hold onto the chain and lower themselves twenty-five to thirty feet till they could grab a handful of mud to prove they touched bottom. The water turned a deeper and deeper green as they dropped down, until it shone emerald.

But this is all secondhand knowledge. Looking back, I realize that I never once spent a summer afternoon at the most popular site in town—or in all of Huntington County. I never swam out to the rocky ledges or dove down to what was left of the old railroad ties. My trips to the quarry were few—and none of them for pleasure.

EMERGENCY CARE

During my second year of medical practice, I was listening to a Chicago White Sox game, when Dorma, the manager of the swimming pool, phoned my home with an urgent request: "Hurry—we have a drowning!"

After Dorma's call it took me only minutes to arrive at the pool and sprint over to a crowd of bathers. Breaking through, I found two lifeguards giving CPR to a boy stretched motionless on the sand. I soon assessed there was no pulse, no spontaneous respirations. The boy's pupils were dilated, indicating his brain wasn't receiving oxygen. We continued giving CPR while the lifeguards explained that this boy must have been underwater for at least twenty minutes.

He was discovered missing at the beginning of a rest period, when a whistle signaled for everyone to leave the water. Each child was supposed to find his or her buddy and then raise their clasped hands. But one swimmer couldn't find his twelve-year-old friend. In fact, no one had seen him for quite some time, and the lifeguards learned he had come to the pool with a neighbor family. The lifeguards immediately swam their gradients, searching for the missing boy. They found him in about five minutes—but never witnessed any movement.

The quarry is spring fed and twenty-six feet deep in the center. This makes the water cold everywhere, except near shore. A cold-water drowning takes longer to occur than one in warm water, but twenty minutes-plus was too long for this boy. We continued CPR as we put him in the ambulance and pulled away, but soon I stopped resuscitation efforts since they were obviously ineffective; there was no evidence of life.

When I spoke with the boy's parents at the hospital, they told me that their son had epilepsy with seizures that were not well controlled. He was not to be swimming unless someone constantly watched him. Most likely, a seizure while underwater had caused his death.

Though this boy was discovered too late to resuscitate, his drowning underscored for me how desperately our community needed an ambulance service with basic equipment and trained personnel. The ambulance that transported the drowned boy was also the mortician's hearse and only offered a small tank of oxygen. I rode in it a number of times during my first two years at Markle. It was different from any ambulance I had ever seen, with the wide door for the stretcher on the right-hand side of the vehicle, instead of in back. When the stretcher was in place, the victim's head rested where the front passenger's seat would normally be. Roe Funderburg preferred this arrangement because when he was transporting someone by himself he could observe and talk with the patient. He told me how he would drive with his left hand and use his right to keep pressure over a bleeding artery or catch vomitus in a container. But this arrangement did not allow room for me to work on a patient during transport, unless I stood behind the driver's seat and reached awkwardly forward.

Over the next year, Lee and I discussed how we could establish an effective ambulance service in Markle. It was a pressing concern. From the summer of 1965 until the following summer, we had thirteen highway fatalities within a four-mile radius of our town. A local family whom Mary and I had grown close to was on their way to the Wells County 4-H Fair when an approaching car ran a stop sign and t-boned their car. William Caley and his children— Kevin (age 8), Kris (11), Kent (12) and Kirby (14)—perished; only Marjorie, the wife and mother, who was ejected into a cornfield, survived. This accident shook our community and matched the 1965 toll for the highest number of deaths in an Indiana highway accident.

More tragedies were on the way. Early one morning eleven-year-old Eddie Espich was fatally struck in Markle while delivering morning newspapers on his bike. That same year a four-year-old girl visiting from Fort Wayne darted into the road and was hit by a car at the east edge of town. For several years, the roads around Markle were closed and routes changed as the Corps of Engineers constructed the Huntington Reservoir and the State Highway Department built Interstate 69. These detours may have contributed to the increased number of traffic accidents as drivers took unfamiliar routes.

One Saturday morning, three ambulances—all from funeral homes—arrived at a two-car accident south of Markle. The ambulance from Markle picked up one patient, since that's all it could hold, and the other two ambulances, both from Huntington, took the remaining patients. One of these ambulances carried four injured passengers. That larger vehicle had two cots that hung from the roof, above two other stretchers. The vehicle's driver stopped by our office because one of the patients on the lower cot complained of severe pain. I could not check him well but assessed that he had a fractured hip and would be all right until he arrived at the emergency room. I asked the other three patients if they were okay, and they seemed to be, but I could not really check them since the ambulance was so stuffed with cots. Later in the morning, I received a phone call from the Fort Wayne Hospital informing me that one of the patients on a top cot was dead upon arrival, apparently from a punctured lung.

Perhaps a better ambulance service would not have made any difference in the deaths of accident victims that year, but when we transported patients in emergency situations we needed to know we were doing everything possible to save their lives.

Markle not only straddles two counties (Huntington and Wells) but contains four townships. For the most part, the township governing units, along with the Town Council, get along well. In 1966, when Lee and I started advancing our idea for an ambulance service linked to the fire department, the township boards were cooperatively financing a well-staffed voluntary fire department headquartered in Markle.

This fire department formed in 1899 when one man was paid six dollars a year to direct volunteers who maneuvered a horse cart equipped with a hundred feet of garden hose. In 1905 the town purchased a single-cylinder compression pump on a cart, and when the fire bell rang, a bucket brigade fed water to the hand-operated pump. In 1928 the department bought its first truck—a new Model A Ford. Throughout the years Markle's fire department maintained a strong reputation for dependability as it fought local and rural fires.

When Lee and I presented our proposal, there was no ambulance service associated with any voluntary fire department in Northeastern Indiana. However, Markle's fire department and administration responded positively to the idea and soon a strong groundswell of support developed. As a first step Lee and I went with the Town Council Chairman and the Fire Department Chief to visit recently established ambulance services run by fire departments in some Indianapolis suburbs. Then we traveled to ambulance dealerships to see our vehicle options. Initially, there were no EMT (Emergency Medical Technician) courses available, so after office hours Lee and I taught the firemen advanced Red Cross First Aid in our waiting room. Later we taught regular EMT classes on how to handle injured patients, assess injuries, keep an open airway, administer oxygen, and perform other basic emergency measures. I greatly enjoyed teaching these courses and felt gratified when I observed how well graduates responded to emergencies within our community.

I rode with many patients on the early ambulance runs. Sometimes I started an intravenous fluid line in our office and continued it on the way to the hospital. At times I administered CPR. I'll never forget the afternoon a nurse and I performed chest compressions on a patient all the way to Lutheran Hospital in Fort Wayne. Lee and I were in the office seeing afternoon patients when we heard a loud thump on the old wooden floorboards. We both rushed toward the receptionist's desk where a man lay on the floor. He wasn't breathing, and he had no heartbeat. Lee and I started CPR with closed chest compressions and mouth-to-mouth resuscitation. As we worked, the receptionist told us that the man was fifty-five years old and had just been making an appointment to see us when he collapsed.

The local ambulance was at the scene within five minutes. While a volunteer fireman pumped oxygen to the patient through an ambu bag mask, Carol Higgins, an RN, helped me apply steady cardiac compressions. In the early 70s, ambulances didn't carry defibrillators, I.V.s, or cardiac medicine, but fortunately, we did have a vehicle large enough for Carol and me to take turns providing the compressions.

When we reached Lutheran, the cardiologist told us we should stop our efforts. "Gerald, they're useless," he said. "The cardiac event happened more than forty-five minutes ago."

I told him that we had been checking the patient's pupils all during the ride and they had always been constricted, indicating his brain was continually receiving oxygen. I said that we must at least try to save him. Though I could tell that the cardiologist was upset by my insistence, he agreed to take over care as the patient was hooked to an EKG monitor, a respiratory resuscitator, and several IVs. When the doctor discovered that the patient was in ventricular fibrillation, he electro-shocked him several times until his heart resumed a normal cardiac rhythm.

Carol and I were exhausted as we rode back to Markle in the ambulance. I wondered whether our patient would live and if he did, whether he'd be mentally sound.

The next day when I stepped into his room he was in bed, attached to many monitors, but alert and breathing on his own. "Why does it hurt so much to breathe?" he asked me. I told him we had broken four ribs on both sides of his chest doing compressions. His recovery was unremarkable except for the healing of his ribs which took about four weeks. Later he had cardiac bypass surgery.

When he did die—many years later—his wife told me it was on the far side of their pond, where he had gone fishing. "I think he knew he was having heart trouble and wanted to be where you could not get to him to break any more ribs," she said.

The new Markle ambulance service became a community endeavor the townspeople took pride in. Doctors and staff at the Fort Wayne hospitals would tell us they knew when patients were brought to them from Markle because they were so well cared for, with preliminary support provided.

Our success in Markle, along with a nation-wide initiative to advance pre-hospital emergency care, stimulated other nearby communities to upgrade their services. I was appointed to the first Northeastern Indiana Emergency Care Commission, an organization that reached out to all the area counties and connected with the national organization. Over the years our emergency medical personnel developed from Basic EMTs to Advanced EMTs to Paramedics who serve from a countywide organization based at the Bluffton hospital with a branch service in Markle and several other small towns.

With all the progress in pre-hospital emergency care, it's hard to believe that once the prevailing philosophy was *load and go* and that the way to *go* was buckled inside a hearse.

THE WOODS

After renting the house on Logan Street for two years, our family moved to another small house in Markle—a plain, white clapboard, just a few blocks away but across the county line on Division Street. This meant that Shari, who had just completed first grade at West Rockcreek School, would be attending East Rockcreek in the fall.

This was the era when school systems all over Indiana were consolidating. Markle's elementary school and high school had closed in the late 1950s, and students now rode buses to one of four rural township schools: West Rockcreek and West Union in Huntington County and East Rockcreek and East Union in Wells County. After learning that Huntington County was planning to construct one huge high school for the entire county and that its new elementary school would be fourteen miles away, Mary and I decided to relocate across the county line so that our children would attend the newly-formed Northern Wells School District, a smaller school corporation and closer to Markle.

Now we lived in a house next door to the Kinzer family, and Shari and Marlis spent many hours with their children— Mark, Mike, Leah, and Matt. They biked around the block together and played home-made versions of TV game shows like Monty Hall's *Let's Make a Deal*. We lived on Division Street for only a year, but it was a year marked by the arrival of our third child, Stephen.

Other doctors who were in partnerships had advised Lee and me to never live beside each other or do many things together, as that would lead to problems among the

83

wives and even the children. But we disregarded this advice. In fact, our families got along so well that Mary and Dawn started looking for larger homes in the area where our growing families could continue living next to each other, houses with yards ample enough for pets, kickball, and tree houses. Eventually, the women discovered an eight-acre woods they felt would be perfect for both families to build in. This woods, along a dirt road just two miles east of Markle, had huge beech, maple, walnut, ash, and locust trees bordered by cornfields. A nearby creek, called Griffin Ditch, meandered toward the Wabash and reminded Mary of the creek near her own childhood farm.

The only complication was that the land wasn't for sale. It was owned by the administrator of the Wells County Hospital, and she didn't really want to sell the woods since it was part of a farm that had been in her family for decades. But no one in her family was still farming, so after some consideration she decided to sell us the woods if we would also buy the surrounding sixteen acres of farmland. That way we'd be taking an even corner from her farm. We agreed to the purchase, and the woodland was divided equally between both families, with the remaining farmland kept in both names.

The woods had thickets of low brush, so before we started building we pastured sheep there. Since sheep favor the taste of poison ivy vines, this was an efficient way to clear that hazard. But our beautiful forest had other dangers—one of which we discovered soon after the sheep began grazing. One evening as our family was exploring the woods, Marlis and Shari came across an old fallen tree. They walked and stomped on it, pretending it was a natural bridge. Suddenly, Mary and I heard screams. A dark cloud had risen from the rotten wood. Hundreds of yellow jackets began chasing the girls as they ran toward us. Grabbing hold of them, we dashed to the car, trying to brush wasps off their hair, arms, legs, and clothes as we ran.

The girls looked pale. I was afraid they might be sensitive to the stings—and who knew how many they had suffered? We drove straight to the office where I planned to give each an injection of adrenaline. But as soon as we entered the empty building, the girls took off. No matter the reason, they didn't want another sting. Marlis was fairly easy to capture since she was only four years old, but Shari was more difficult. Fortunately, Lee happened to drop in during the chase and I let him administer the injections. Back home, as Mary helped the girls undress, dead yellow jackets fell from even their underclothes.

Later that summer, after Mossburg Construction had finished staking the boundaries for our homes and was preparing to excavate the basements, two men entered the office and introduced themselves as surveyors for the Indiana Department of Natural Resources. They said they had heard we were planning to build homes in an area that would be a flood plain for the new Huntington Reservoir. They were currently surveying about two miles east of our woods. As they came west, anything below a nine-hundred-and-four-foot elevation would be labeled a flood plain, with new buildings prohibited.

Lee and I felt devastated to think that our plans for a home in the woods would fall apart. But then, sensing our disappointment, one of the surveyors had an idea. "We won't arrive at your property for another week," he said.

"Before we do, you could build a dike along your land, and when we reach it, we'll be able to just skirt the woods. To get the dirt for this dike, you could dig yourself a pond, and then you'd have a place to fish and swim."

I loved this idea and so did Lee. We appreciated how thoughtful someone could be, even when there was nothing in it for him. We called our wives to get their approval and then phoned the excavators who were poised with their bulldozers to carve out our basements. Instead, they built us a long dike that week and dug a one-acre pond that later became our swimming hole in summer and ice skating rink in winter. Over the years it harbored large catfish who'd surface for bread crumbs when they heard us clapping our hands. Mallards used the pond and so did foxes and deer that would edge down for a drink. Along the dike we planted white pine that in fifteen years grew to form a windbreak.

Soon after we moved into our new homes, we heard a holler for help from the northeast. "Help! Help! Help!" a voice shrieked, but all of the Millers and Kinzers were accounted for. Mary and I thought maybe one of our neighbors who lived across the railroad tracks about a quarter mile away was in trouble. So she and I started driving with the windows rolled down, and, sure enough, as we drove, the calls grew louder. Pulling into the driveway of a house where two elderly sisters lived, we soon saw the source of the urgent cry: two peacocks perched on a shed roof, their cupped tail feathers catching the late afternoon light as they hollered for a house call they clearly didn't need.

Eventually, we grew accustomed to the peacocks and to the freight trains that rumbled past. We marveled at all the interesting sounds in the woods, especially at night: the *Who cooks for you? Who cooks for you all?* of the barred owl, the cheep of tree frogs, the sharp yap of young foxes along the dike.

Perhaps what I liked best about living in the woods was being near lots of animals again. During my boyhood I spent much of my time caring for farm animals and figured that one day I'd be a veterinarian. However, when pre-medicine and pre-veterinary students were grouped together during my freshman year at Goshen College, I became exposed to the medical field and realized that my goal had changed, that I was more interested in the health problems of people. But I still enjoyed animals and so did the Kinzers, so both sides of the woods quickly filled up with pets.

My family's first and most beloved pet was an intelligent Scotch collie named Lady. Lady recognized the cars of our friends and wouldn't make a sound when they drove up. But if an unfamiliar car parked at the end of our long drive or close to the house, we knew her bark meant we should check out the stranger.

One afternoon when Mary was alone, she heard Lady barking but didn't see anything unusual until she opened the garage door. A young man stood on the driveway, facing her. "Ma'am, I'm selling encyclopedias to work my way through college," he said. "I'd like to tell you about them."

"I'm sorry, we already have a set," Mary said.

The man started giving reasons why she should buy his books anyway. When Mary still declined to consider buying, he started cussing. Meanwhile, Lady had been watching the man intently. When the man's face grew red and he shook his fist at Mary, shouting, "You don't want me to go to college!" Lady leapt between her and the salesman, barking and growling. "Get back to your mama!" the man cried as he jumped on his bike and sped off, with Lady snapping at his heels all the way to the mailbox.

One day an elderly horse trader who had come to the office for a routine appointment said to me, "I have the horse for you. He's a five-year-old Appaloosa." This man had a small farm near Huntertown where he stabled the horses he traded and the ones he kept for city dwellers in Fort Wayne. This small horse was well-trained, he said, and would be just right for my children. As a boy, I had enjoyed my own pony, so I told him that on the weekend we'd take a look at his horse. That, of course, was tantamount to saying, "I'll buy him," because when the kids saw the horse they immediately wanted him.

Even with Shari feeding and brushing this horse, there was more work than I anticipated. Horses have to be fed and watered and then that means manure to be shoveled. The old barn across the road was easy to prepare, but I needed to fence in part of the field for a pasture.

Pinho, whose Portuguese name originated from a Brazilian exchange student living with us at the time, did prove to be a good horse, his only bad habits being a tendency to expand his stomach while being saddled, graze on grass when urged to move forward, and rub against trees. But all a rider had to do was spur Pinho in the direction of the barn and he took off as if he'd received a shot of adrenalin.

At one time or another, we also raised rabbits, lambs, and various fowl. In the barn across the road, we boarded a peacock for a friend and had our own fancy bantam chickens and ducks. Once, when one of the ducks was injured by a neighbor's dog, I decided the humane thing to do would be to put her out of her misery. Shari was not so sure about this, but she could see the duck's agony. Her wing was broken and she hobbled around, eyes glazed with pain. I promised Shari that the death would be quick, and she went with me to dig a deep grave so no dog or coyote would dig up the body.

As a boy, I was accustomed to butchering chickens, but the task of chopping off heads always fell to my father who was quick with the hatchet. Now it was my turn. Shari held the duck as I gripped the axe handle and, fortunately, severed the head with one stroke. The body flopped some but then lay still. I positioned the duck in her grave, covered her with dirt, and then started to pack the dirt by stamping. But each time I stomped, we heard a quack.

This voice from underground indicated that a duck's voice originates deeper down than its throat and, more importantly, it seemed to contradict the assurance I'd given earlier—that the duck would die quickly. It was a terrible thing, like the tell-tale heart in Poe's story, to hear that mallard quack and quack as I buried her, seemingly alive.

As a general rule, Mary wasn't much attached to our domestic animals (except for Lady). Her favorite creatures in the woods were the songbirds—cardinals and goldfinches and especially the Jenny wrens that nested near the house. Every spring Mary's ear was tuned to catch the first low notes of their warbling songs. She favored hummingbirds, too, and lured them to the yard with salvia, coral bells, fushia, bee balm, red hot pokers, and lobelia.

A lot of the wild animals in our woods—like the raccoons beneath our deck and the chipmunks in our basement walls—seemed fairly at ease with us. But sometimes I thought about the wild creatures that hadn't been able to co-exist with the early settlers—animals that had been hunted to extinction in the area, like cougars, bears, wolves, and passenger pigeons. In the 1800s, millions of passenger pigeons roosted in Wells County and feasted on the abundant beechnuts and acorns. As flocks approached they'd sound like distant thunder, and as they passed overhead, their bodies darkened the sun. These birds that threatened farmers' crops were shot for sport or food or for the oil that was rendered from their bodies.

Wolves would have roamed our woods and rattlesnakes, too. Both were sacred animals for the Miami who had a village near Markle, at the confluence of the Wabash and Rock Creek. Rattlesnakes, *cicikwia*, were especially venerated, and the Miami left them tobacco offerings near their dens in the river bluffs near Huntington. But the settlers had an understandable fear of rattlesnake venom and held huge snake-killings each spring that depleted their numbers. When the snakes, still lethargic from hibernation, slid out of their dens to sun themselves on rocks, men and boys sealed up the entrances and clubbed the snakes with spades and crowbars. From the fattest snakes, they extracted oil to make a medicine for rheumatism.

Eventually, almost all of the forest was chopped down and the mosquito-infested wetlands were drained. There were no more wolves to attack young calves or colts. No more passenger pigeons to damage a crop. No poisonous snakebites or deaths from malaria. But there was also not much wilderness left. Bordered by corn and bean fields, only pockets of woodland remained—tightly wedged remnants like ours and the long narrow bands along creeks and the river.

We kept the back section of our woods in a natural state, but other areas we cleared of underbrush to add flowering bushes, such as lilac and mock orange, and small trees like redbud and mountain ash. I enjoyed yard work and found the grip of a shovel or a rake a nice contrast to handling a stethoscope or syringe. Because of time restrictions, I seldom golfed, but I could take time to mow a section of the yard, plant bulbs, trim the forsythia bushes, or burn autumn leaves. As the poet May Sarton wrote, "Everything that slows us down and forces patience, everything that sets us back into the slow circles of nature, is a help. Gardening is an instrument of grace."

Mary and I never regretted that we built next to the Kinzers. Laurel and Lynn Kinzer were born after the move, and nine children were enough for a game of whiffle ball or kick ball or an evening of kick-the-can. Our children climbed trees together, pedaled their bikes around the circular drive, and coasted downhill to the creek. In winter both families gathered at the pond for bonfires and ice skating; in summer we broke from our yard work to just talk. We proved the naysayers wrong and dubbed our woods, "Pair-o'-docs."

THREE: FROM MY MEDICAL BAG

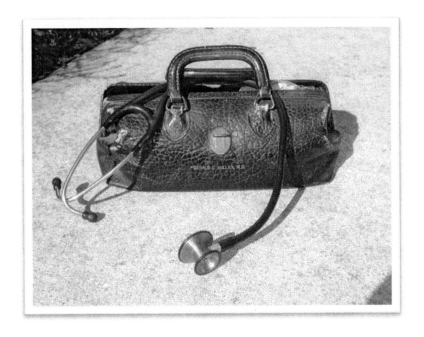

EMBLEM OF THE TRADE

In one of my favorite Norman Rockwell paintings, *Doctor and Doll*, a white-haired physician is seated at a roll-top desk with the bell of his stethoscope against the chest of a doll a girl holds forward. The girl's face bears a concerned expression while the doctor, with his head tilted for concentration, has a twinkle in his eye. On the floor near his feet lies an emblem of his profession—a black medical bag.

At the end of my second year of medical school as I was entering the clinical phase of training, the Eli Lilly Company gave me and each of my classmates one such shiny black bag, each with our initials. Gripping the handle, I had the sense that one day soon I would finally be a real doctor.

I used that bag for decades until the handle grew torn and the sides lost their sheen. It was always with me, either by my side or in the car. A stethoscope and blood pressure cuff were its most useful contents—though, more often than not, the stethoscope was not inside the bag, but around my neck. Since I used this instrument so much, it seemed handier to keep it out of the bag, though my son says I had an ulterior motive.

Whenever I've gotten on his case for a speeding ticket, Steve has had a favorite response: "Dad, you never got tickets because you always drove with a stethoscope around your neck so the police would think you were going to an emergency." That might have been true—on a subconscious level. Sometimes on the way to the hospital I would notice that I was being followed, but when I'd pull into the hospital parking lot, the patrol car would veer off. More likely than not, the local police recognized my car, rather than took note of my stethoscope. One of the doctors who eventually joined our staff—Dr. Marcelo Gavilaniz, an obstetrician—used his stethoscope to optimal advantage. When he needed to rush to the hospital for a delivery, he'd wave it out the window to any police officer who might observe him speeding or running a red light with no one coming.

In addition to a blood pressure cuff—and a stethoscope in absentia—my black bag held an otoscope for checking ears, an ophthalmoscope for observing the back of the eyes, and a percussion hammer and tuning fork for doing neurological examinations. It also contained a package of sterile gloves, a packet of wooden tongue depressors, a tube of K-Y lubricating jelly, and from time to time a few other supplies.

This small black bag helped me to diagnosis the problems on house calls or emergencies, but for treatment I carried a larger, box-like bag—my medicine bag. Actually, I own several medicine bags; the others are gifts from patients whose relatives were doctors. One from the 20s or 30s has rows of tiny vials filled with medicines in powder or pill form: aspirin, antacids, bile salt, milk of magnesia, and other items that today are bought across the counter. But some of the vials contain strychnine, as well as mercuric chloride, powdered digitalis, and oil of juniper. Larger bottles hold quinine, camphor, and extract of belladonna. I would venture to guess that it was usually not this bag's powder and pills that healed patients, but the compassionate care of its owner—or the curative power of time.

The contents in my own medicine bag changed dramatically through the years. At first, one of the standard antibiotics I carried was penicillin, but I eliminated that after a harrowing after-hours visit with the pastor of a rural church near Markle.

"I'm coming down with a bad sore throat and starting to get a cough," the reverend said over the phone. "I have to preach a sermon tomorrow and can't afford to lose my voice. Would you see me and maybe give me a shot so what I have won't get worse?"

We met at the office where I examined him as we chatted. When I asked if he was allergic to any medicine, he said that he wasn't. While we continued talking, I decided to give him an injection of penicillin and then put him on penicillin tablets and a decongestant.

As soon as I gave him the injection, my patient said, "I hope you didn't give me penicillin. I had an injection of that when I was in the army and nearly died." Soon the pastor was looking pale and having difficulty breathing. His skin was clammy. He felt nauseated.

I laid him down and reached for the adrenalin and the hydrocortisone that we always had available in the office for acute allergic reactions. I continued talking with him as I administered nasal oxygen from the nearby tank. My patient never lost consciousness, but his blood pressure plummeted to almost zero before he started breathing more easily and regained his color.

I stayed with him for about an hour as he returned to normal. I told him that he needed to always tell medical personnel that he had a penicillin allergy and that in case he was in an accident and unconscious, he also needed to wear a tag around his neck that identified his allergy. My patient drove home, but I called him later in the evening and the next morning to check on him. He said he was fine and that he didn't even have a sore throat or a cough.

After that, Lee and I removed the penicillin vials from our medical bags. If I had given the pastor an injection at his home and driven away, he surely would have died.

Over time, Ampicillin and Tetracycline also disappeared from my bag as I made fewer house calls on children and as more antibiotics became available. In general, I relied more on my prescription pad. As I began going to high school athletic events, I started carrying more suture supplies and bandages. I frequently needed to stitch a chin or forehead so an injured football or basketball player could get back in the game. I also started carrying syringes and tubes to collect blood and cultures as more of my house calls were to the elderly, housebound, or disabled.

I wanted to be prepared for emergencies so I stored a small oxygen tank and a face mask in my car trunk, along with oral airways of varying sizes. In my medicine bag, I carried nitroglycerine tablets, an injectable diuretic (Lasix), and Lanoxin for acute cardiac episodes. In case I needed to treat an acute asthmatic, I had injectable medicines. One September night the ragweed pollen count rose so high that numerous patients called, wanting an injection. In fact, so many called that I started telling them to come to my home. Eventually, a line of cars extended all around our circular drive. Over time, as preventative medicines improved, I didn't need to see asthmatics as emergencies. I also didn't need to treat patients with acute migraine headaches since medicines were developed that either prevented these headaches or controlled them at the onset.

In 1950, Dr. William Gordan wrote in *GP* that the black medical bag has "represented many things . . . ranging from the contemptuous belief that it contained only evil smelling and tasting concoctions of little value at one extreme, to the open-mouthed, awe-inspired belief of children in days gone by who were told that it was the receptacle from which new baby brothers and sisters were plucked." To me, the black medical bag represents a doctor's willingness to go wherever he or she is needed—by horse, car, snowmobile, or foot.

Now that I'm retired, my little black bag and my medicine bag are in my basement, just artifacts in a small medical museum I've pulled together. They're on a shelf next to a rectal ether machine and other antiques.

EPIDEMICS

Markle's cemetery spans a hillside above the Wabash River. It's a graveyard without large trees, exposed to the brunt of winter's cold or summer's heat. For the most part, the gray stones lie low to the ground and lack distinction. The unusual names, however, echo across the expanse of time—*Lemuel, Leander, Sylvanus* and *Isham; Clellah, Vernecia, Alpha* and *Coola*. And in the oldest section of the cemetery, where names are only faint indentations, the markers tilt on time's edge, like ships caught in a frozen sea.

I read the footnotes of history by wandering between the rows. Infectious outbreaks have carved their dates on some of the older stones. Before the development of vaccines, virulent infections like poliomyelitis, measles, Asian flu, Asiatic cholera, small pox, typhoid, and diphtheria struck Markle and the surrounding communities with brutal force, often taking the very young and the very old. I remember Verna Seibold Stockman telling me about a diphtheria epidemic that spread through Markle in 1910. Diphtheria is a bacterial disease with an incubation period of one week and symptoms that include a sore throat, fever, swollen lymph nodes, and the formation over the tonsils and pharynx of a thick, grayish membrane that interferes with breathing and swallowing. This disease can also affect the heart, kidneys, and nervous system. Verna, who was born in 1884 and had a clear memory even in her nineties, told me that during the diphtheria outbreak people were afraid to leave their homes. With almost every family losing at least one member, about ten percent of the townspeople died.

Frank S. Bash records that an earlier epidemic of Asiatic cholera almost depopulated the young settlement of Huntington in 1849. Thirty-two people died within twenty-four hours of coming down with the first symptoms. Businesses closed and people fled to the country. Five years later, the epidemic returned and twenty-eight Huntington residents died, as well as a hundred laborers who were laying tracks for the Wabash Railway. Charles Follett, a man from Ohio who was engaged to a Huntington woman, arrived in town on a Wednesday for his marriage, took sick with cholera on Friday night at his hotel, died on Saturday, and was buried on Sunday, the same day he and his fiancée had planned to be wed.

John Kenower of Huntington was an undertaker during both epidemics. "I witnessed some desperate scenes," he wrote. "I have seen men drawn up almost in a knot, every muscle in the body twitching, and with a cry of pain the man was dead. They usually took sick in the morning and died the following evening or took sick in the evening and died the next morning. They lay around, some of them on the ground, dying like flies. I hauled them by loads to the cemetery, but have no idea how many I buried altogether." Until the sulfa drugs were available in the 1930s and penicillin in the early '40s, Huntington and Wells County residents did not have much recourse when epidemics hit but to close the schools and rely on folk remedies.

In *Wells County Towns and Townships: A Pictorial History*, Barbara Elliott writes that schools in the area frequently closed their doors during outbreaks of flu, smallpox, diphtheria, and even tonsillitis. This was a good precaution, especially since students usually drank from a common water bucket, using the same tin cup or long-handled dipper. Elliott writes that during epidemics, popular folk medicine included "a bag of asafetida tied around the neck, a stink bug tied in a thimble, an onion poultice, or turpentine and lard, all of which served to keep others away if nothing else." Asafetida (also called devil's dung) was a bitter and foul-smelling resinous gum made from the roots of giant fennel. It was believed to be potent at warding off germs by absorbing them. Elliott mentions that "rail fences along the way to school made good storage places for the asafetida bags during the day with the bags being picked up near home in the evening."

Due to the 1918 Spanish Flu pandemic, schools in the Markle area were shut down that year, and if you go to area cemeteries, you will find a disproportionate number of stones with the date of death inscribed as 1918 or 1919. Many of the graves belong to women of child-bearing age. Doctors have an adage about who will be most acutely affected by flu epidemics: "the very young, the very old, the very ill, and the very pregnant." During the 1918 pandemic only the last part of that saying held true. In fact, for some unknown reason, the mortality rate was highest among adults twenty to fifty years old.

When the Hong Kong Flu of 1968-69 hit, it was the first epidemic I dealt with as a doctor. Our daily patient count at the office soared to well over a hundred. Lee and I cancelled many routine appointments as we assessed the severely ill and those needing antibiotics for secondary infections. Which child was developing pneumonia? Who was becoming dehydrated? Such questions preoccupied my mind as I worried that I might overlook some ill patient who needed more intensive care.

Our hospital had a capacity of thirty-three beds, but during the peak of the epidemic we squeezed fifty or more into the rooms, hallways, and even the visitors' lounge. The nursing staff worked hard to provide some sense of privacy for each patient, and retired nurses came back to help with the increased workload. Lee and I made rounds twice each day to be sure we were doing everything we could for each flu victim. Worldwide, this epidemic killed over one million people, but with better supportive care and antibiotics, our country did not see a high mortality rate.

When we started practice, fear of contagion from childhood diseases was strong and Lee and I either saw children infected with these illnesses in their homes or ushered them through the back door of the office to wait in a separate examining room. Until the introduction of a vaccine in 1963, measles accounted for five to ten thousand deaths each year in the United States and seventeen thousand cases of mental retardation. In 1971 I was thankful we gained the MMR vaccine which gave us a way of preventing measles, mumps, and rubella.

I once saw a child die from chickenpox encephalitis. That was when I was an intern. I realized then that chickenpox is not always the innocuous disease that many people think causes only discomfort. Before the chickenpox (varicella) vaccine became available in 1995, more than eleven thousand children were hospitalized each year in the U.S. and about a hundred died. Some mothers would ask what I thought about going to "pox parties," gatherings where mothers would bring their children to be exposed to another child who had chickenpox so as to get the disease out of the way. I recommended against going to these, cautioning that the disease should not be taken lightly — that isolation and a vaccine would be more prudent.

Although prudence is sensible, it is not wise to live in fear. We will probably never be free of the threat of epidemics, but from day to day, our bodies reveal an astonishing capacity for healing. As the American physician and essayist Lewis Thomas once wrote, "The great secret of doctors, known only to their wives, but still hidden from the public, is that most things get better by themselves, most things, in fact, are better in the morning."

POLIO

While growing up in the 1940s and early '50s, my sisters and I had the chickenpox, the mumps, and three types of measles. My older sister, Jewel, also had scarlet fever which quarantined all of us for fourteen days. We had no complications from these viral infections, but each caused us soreness or itching for seven to nine days. Our real fear, and the fear of our parents, was that we might develop polio. My cousin, Donnie, died of poliomyelitis when he was a sophomore in high school, and I knew others who were paralyzed or died from the disease or its complications. News reports kept updating us on the number of Hoosiers dying each year from polio. My parents strictly forbade me or my sisters to swim in August, eat apples sprayed with pesticides, or join large crowds because they had heard that all of these things might be related to catching that dreaded disease.

The year 1954 when I was sixteen was a peak year for poliomyelitis in Indiana. One thousand, four hundred and forty-eight cases were reported and most occurred to people under the age of twenty. Fortunately, Jonas Salk's new vaccine was licensed the next year and mass inoculation began. Nationwide, the incidence of polio decreased from thirty-five thousand cases in 1953 to only a hundred and sixty-one cases ten years later. In 1954, when Salk was asked who owned the patent to his vaccine, he quipped, "The people, I would say. There is no patent. Could you patent the sun?" It was a great relief to me that by the time I began my practice in Markle this vaccine was credited for wiping out polio in Indiana.

Fifteen years earlier, in 1949, Dr. Woods had diagnosed one of my patients, Howard Best, with polio. Howard spent ten weeks at St. Joe Hospital in Fort Wayne, acquiring an exercise routine that helped him move his arms and legs. His wife, Kathryn, learned to drive their Plymouth so she could visit him. Between trips, she handled the farm chores and cared for their two young sons. When Howard returned home, the corn still needed to be harvested, but it wasn't long until forty men driving eighteen tractors with corn pickers came down the road. Thirty-two women cooked food for the workers.

That year Howard devised his own physical therapy: he learned to operate a sewing machine and in one year made eighty aprons. His brother built an exercise rail that hung above his bed, and a friend loaned him a parachute harness that served as a bed lift. Eventually, Howard learned to walk again and to drive a tractor by sitting on a boat-winch platform.

As a new doctor I knew I'd be treating the long-term effects of polio on survivors but chances were slim that I would ever diagnose a new case. An experience during my internship, however, taught me that I always needed to be alert to what might contradict my assumptions.

One Sunday afternoon in 1963 I was called to the emergency room at Lutheran to see a twelve-year-old boy from Warsaw, a city thirty-five miles away. This boy had been sick for about ten days, and his condition was worsening. The illness started with a cold and a sore neck that eventually became stiff and weak. Now the boy's extremities were also extremely weak; he was short of breath and unable to hold up his head without support. His parents reported that they had been taking him to their family doctor, a chiropractor, who had given their son daily cervical adjustments.

This doctor had been unavailable for the past three days, and that Sunday their son was so much weaker that he was having trouble swallowing and breathing. The emergency room in Warsaw sent him immediately to our hospital, and when he arrived, I called the pediatrician on call for emergencies, an experienced doctor in his sixties. He told me over the phone that he thought this child had polio even though there had been no acute cases in Indiana in over five years. Dr. Bash then came immediately to the hospital and confirmed the diagnosis. He said the boy had bulbar polio, the worse type since it involved the brainstem of the spinal column, thereby affecting the boy's breathing and swallowing.

Most iron lung machines had long been dismantled, but Dr. Bash remembered that some were stored in the basement of St. Joseph Hospital. Emergency crews worked hard, and within three hours we had our patient sedated and resting comfortably in a working iron lung. At first the machine only assisted his breathing, but within twenty-four hours it was doing the breathing for him. There was no medicine to help treat polio, so all we could do was support our patient as his body fought the disease.

The boy's condition continued to deteriorate. Within three days, he could not speak with us. I would visit several times each day, talking to him but not knowing if he understood. There was just the rhythmical bellow of the iron lung, eighteen times a minute—the positive pressure and then the negative pressure, making his chest expand and then deflate. I saw the wild look in this child's eyes—the intense fear.

We gave him intravenous fluids and after several days placed a nasal feeding tube into his stomach for nutrition. At first he could wiggle his fingers and toes, but at the end of a week there were no voluntary movements. During the last days of his life, it was difficult to tell if he was even alive, but we could hear a faint heartbeat each time we turned off his iron lung to check his condition. After eighteen days in the hospital, he died.

We were heartbroken that we were not able to save this young life. I felt worse when I heard from the family that on the advice of their chiropractor they had refused to give any of their children the polio vaccine. That doctor was blind, having lost his vision several years earlier. Perhaps if he could have seen from one day to the next how ill his patient was becoming, he might have called for medical assistance.

To the best of my knowledge, this child's illness was the last documented case of bulbar polio in the state of Indiana.

ALTERNATIVE MEDICINE

In 1913, when Alfreda Mossburg was three years old, she heard her Aunt Nora tell her mom, "You'd better try it because that kid looks awfully peaked!" The aunt was referring to the folk cure for stunted growth called *measuring*.

In order to have Alfreda measured, her mother and aunt took her to Mary Keller, a "string doctor" who lived in Markle. When they arrived, the two women had to remain upstairs while Alfreda was measured for "short growth" in the basement. This was because a man could observe a woman taking measurements or a woman could observe a man taking them, but the same sex was never allowed to watch. "She used a piece of string," Alfreda remembers in her memoir *Journey into Yesterday*, "and measured me up and down and sideways, around my head and down my arms and legs."

According to Wayland Debs Hand in *Magical Medicine: The Folkloric Component of Medicine in the Folk Belief, Custom, and Ritual of the People of Europe and America*, the first recorded practice of measuring someone to discover and cure an illness goes all the way back to Pliny the Elder in the first century A.D. In addition to helping resolve growth problems, measuring has been used for many other illnesses, including madness and even wife-beating. In the first decades of the twentieth century, parents in Indiana and all over the U.S. frequently took their undersized or oversized children to see a string doctor. If the child's length was not seven times the length of his or her foot, the child was diagnosed with short growth. If the length was longer, then he had long growth. Sometimes the diagnosis was based on the ratio of body length to arm span. If height and arm span were equivalent, then the child was normal. During the measuring process, carefully guarded magical words ensured the illness was transferred from the child to the string. Afterward, parents were told to tie the string to a gate post, a grindstone, or maybe a buggy axle—some place where it would be worn through quickly. As soon as the string broke, the healing process could begin.

Mary Keller told Alfreda's mother to wind the string around the singletree on the buggy and that when it wore in two, her daughter would start to grow. With her characteristic sense of irony and good humor, Alfreda admitted, "It worked after about twelve years, for then I became a dumpling and have remained one ever since."

When I came to Markle, a folk cure for warts was still being practiced, but instead of using string, it utilized thread. Norma Steinhilber, Shari's kindergarten teacher, would wrap a thread around someone's wart and then have that person put the thread in a place where it could wear down. When it wore through, the wart would begin to disappear.

"Burn doctors" who could relieve the pain of scorched skin also lived in the Markle area. Janice Jordan, our nurse, told me that when she was an aide at Huntington Hospital a woman who worked there was known for "blowing out fires." When burn patients were admitted, this woman was called up from the kitchen to help ease the pain. No one could watch what she did—but traditionally the art of blowing out burns has involved repeating a bible verse and touching the burn.

A receptionist at our office, Janice Spahr, told me that years ago a Mrs. McBride was Markle's burn doctor. Janice remembered she treated a boy for pain after he fell into a washtub of scalding water. Unfortunately, the boy's burns were so severe that he died.

Zanesville resident Etta Smuts was still *blowing out burns* when I first came to Markle. She also practiced *blood stopping*, another folk cure. Marlene Hoopingarner, a secretary and receptionist in our office, told me that Etta treated her father after he came home from having polyps removed from his nose. "Once he was home, his nose wouldn't stop bleeding," Marlene said. "He asked Mom to take him to Mrs. Smuts' house and she performed 'whatever' to Dad. Right then, his nose stopped bleeding. Mrs. Smuts supposedly did pass on her secrets to another person, though I don't know who, only that the person was a man."

Studies reveal that a patient's state of mind can affect the healing process. Though such folk cures as measuring and blowing out burns have no medicinal value per se, their efficacy may be in the faith patients have in the healer and also in the community support they feel when such healing rituals are performed.

Folk medicine was disappearing by the time I arrived at Markle, but my patients were sometimes attracted to other, more modern forms of alternative medicine.

One of my first house calls was to a farmhouse to see an elderly farmer who was having a lot of low back pain and difficulty walking due to pain in his right hip. I asked if he had been to another doctor and if he had any x-rays. The patient's daughter, a chiropractor, said they had the diagnosis of prostate cancer and that it had spread to his bones. His radiation treatments hadn't helped much and the pain was getting worse. Doctors had given them no other suggestions.

"Would you give our father injections of Krebiozen if we could obtain them?" she asked. I had heard about this drug. It was developed by Dr. Stevan Durovic, who claimed the substance was prepared from the blood of horses injected with bacteria, and promoted by Dr. Andrew Conway Ivy in Chicago. But I also knew Krebiozen had been denounced by the American Medical Association and taken off the market. The family said they could buy it on the black market in Gary, Indiana and insisted they wanted to try it. I thought about the situation for some time and then told the family that I was not recommending Krebiozen, but because nothing else seemed to be available for treatment, I would get syringes for them and demonstrate how to give the medicine.

The drug they obtained came in an unmarked bottle with a paper indicating how much to give and the frequency of injections. I gave the patient his first injection and showed the daughter how to give future ones. Her father's condition grew worse so I started prescribing him stronger pain medication and later injectable narcotics. His family was appreciative that I helped them with the Krebiozen, even though it had proven useless. They felt they had at least tried everything they could. A few months later I heard that Dr. Ivy and his associates had been indicted for fraud, as there was nothing in the liquid but mineral oil and creatine monohydrate, an amino acid found in muscle tissue and sold as a dietary supplement.

Defined by the National Science Foundation as "all treatments that have not been proven effective using scientific methods," alternative medicine presents a dilemma to physicians who must decide what approach to take toward it in their practice. Patients often feel like there should be a treatment for every disease and that they need to try something when conventional medicine has little or nothing to offer.

Soon after setting up practice, I discovered that some of my cancer patients were disappearing for weeks at a time. Gradually, I learned they were going to Mexico to get Laetrile, also called Vitamin B17, a chemically modified form of amygdalin, a substance found in almonds and the pits of apricots and peaches. I wouldn't see the patients with slow-growing cancers for several months, but those with fast-growing tumors I'd see again soon because of their pain. I learned not to be critical of these patients who were grasping for any hope available. Typically, they returned from Mexico, not only with Laetrile, but with sacks of medication of all kinds, part of a "metabolic therapy," that included digestive enzymes, immuno-stimulants, megavitamins, and minerals.

The patients also brought back the sure expectation they would be healed. Even when Laetrile was obviously failing, they found reasons not to blame the treatment. One thirty-eight-year-old mother, whose metastatic breast cancer had spread to her liver and bone, told me: "I know I'd be cured if only I could take all this medicine, but I am so sick I can only get a few pills down each day." I counted thirty different bottles of medicine, and from many of the bottles, she was to take two to six pills daily. These pills gave her hope, but it was a false hope. Some types of cancer have a slow progression with periods of exacerbation and regression. Patients taking Laetrile would often credit the drug for an initial improvement which was actually a natural stage in the disease.

Although most people in Indiana went to Mexico to obtain Laetrile, some found U.S. doctors who sold it. One day I was asked to consult with an older woman concerned for her forty-year-old niece, a patient of mine with a long-standing history of seizures who had just learned she also had diabetes. Her aunt wanted me to convince her that she should go with her to get Laetrile therapy for these diseases. "Why do you feel so strongly about Laetrile therapy?" I asked.

"I had colon cancer five years ago and Laetrile completely cured me," she answered.

I then asked how the cancer was diagnosed and if the doctor had done a biopsy or surgical removal.

"I had some bleeding from my rectum on a Friday," she replied, "and on Monday I went to a doctor who gave me Laetrile. Nobody looked in my rectum, and I had no surgery. I just know that I had cancer and I was cured. They even published my testimonial as a newspaper advertisement." I tried to reason with her, to convince her that we were controlling her niece's epilepsy and could also control her diabetes, that she was not a candidate for Laetrile, but the woman wouldn't budge in her conviction. I knew there was no chance I could convince her that she never had cancer and that the bleeding was probably from a ruptured hemorrhoid.

The use of an alternative medicine is understandable when there is no effective treatment for a disease and the faith it engenders may be helpful to the healing process. The danger occurs when a patient opts for an alternative medicine when a scientifically-proven medicine is available.

One of my patients was a man in his sixties who suffered from hypertension. I had been seeing him for almost twenty years when one morning he was brought by ambulance to the hospital emergency room. He was paralyzed on his right side and confused, with difficulty speaking. His blood pressure was extremely high—280/140. I knew he was having a stroke, one that started at least four hours before he arrived.

I told his wife that I was surprised his blood pressure was so high because I thought we had it well-controlled by several different medications.

She replied, "My husband was tired of taking those pills and they were expensive. He heard that if he took garlic pills they would cure his high blood pressure. So he stopped his medicine and has been taking garlic for a couple of weeks."

Medical articles from the early 1900s tout the benefits of garlic for hypertension, but effective medicine was not available then—not until the 1940s. I don't know if garlic has any effect on blood pressure, but, if it does, it is so minute that it should never be a substitute for the medicines we now have. I told those who wanted to try it to go ahead—as long as they never stopped or reduced their blood pressure medicine. My patient did not die from his stroke, but for the next six years, until his death, he lived handicapped and mostly in a nursing home.

Many herbal remedies, like garlic, are not considered a medicine and so are not controlled by any agency. Anyone can recommend an herb, and anyone can make an herbal treatment and sell it. Some plant extracts do, of course, have medicinal value. For example, digitalis comes from foxglove and has been well-known for two hundred years as a heart medication, though now the synthetic version is safer and more effective. Other plant extracts like quinine and Taxol also have important medicinal properties. We need to keep studying plants for potential cures, but I found it tragic when my patients with diseases that needed medical care delayed diagnosis and treatment while they tried ineffective herbal cures. It was also sad to see patients who had trouble affording the medicines I prescribed go on an expensive regimen of useless megavitamins and herbs.

Some of these patients went to an Amish herbalist in a neighboring county who did not call himself a doctor, as he only had an eighth-grade education, but let other people call him that. This man had an office in the corner of his barn, behind a curtain, and diagnosed patients by looking into their eyes, noting patterns, colors, and irregularities that corresponded to the health of different tissues and organs. *Iridology*, the name of the alternative medicine technique he practiced, goes back several hundred years. A description of iridological principles was first published in the seventeenth century, and the first use of the term *Augendiagnostik*, "eye-diagnosis," was by a nineteenth-century Hungarian doctor, Ignaz von Peczely, who noticed that streaks in the eye of a patient he was treating for a broken leg matched streaks in the eye of an owl whose leg the physician had broken many years earlier.

Patients would come back to me after a trip to the Amish iridologist and say, "He looked in my eyes and immediately knew what was wrong with me." They might say, "He told me my knees hurt and they do hurt." Or, "He told me that I have gallbladder disease with a lot of gas, and I do have a lot of gas." I'm sure this man was uncommonly observant and could tell a lot about a patient's health just by watching his or her movements and demeanor.

Like the doctors who measured or blew out a burn, he never charged for an examination. String doctors like Mary Keller believed that their healing power came from God and that if they asked for money, their gift would leave them. This may have been true for the iridologist, but he also knew that if he asked for payment he would have been vulnerable to the allegation of practicing medicine without a license. He did provide a basket for donations and sold the herbs he prescribed.

TUMORS

One of my first patients was an elderly woman who asked me for pain medication. "Aspirin isn't taking care of my chest pain. I need something stronger," she said. "The pain is so bad that I can't sleep at night."

I noticed an unpleasant odor emanating from her and said she needed to unbutton her blouse so that I could examine her chest.

The woman hesitated, saying, "I just need pain pills." Reluctantly, though, she complied, revealing a chest wrapped in bandages. Beneath these bandages, the right breast had a lump the size of a baseball. It was draining bloody and purulent secretions onto dressings made from gauze padding and strips of old dresses. She said that the nurse and I were the only ones who knew she had this tumor. She hadn't wanted to worry her husband and children.

This woman's breast cancer might not have been fatal if only she would have sought medical treatment when she first found the growth. But in the early '60s we had nothing except supportive assistance to offer patients with such advanced cancer.

In the first twenty years of our practice we scheduled many mastectomies. For patients with invasive tumors we would also order post-surgical radiation treatments. For those not cured, hormonal manipulation might be beneficial for an indefinite period of time. Looking back at those early operations, I imagine how anxious these women must have been as they were wheeled into surgery for a lump in their breast, not knowing until they woke up whether it was benign or malignant, whether they'd have a small scar and a drain in place or would be missing their breast, most of the lymph nodes in their axilla, and some of their chest muscles.

One Sunday evening in my first year of practice, a local man called, asking if I would see his wife who was in severe pain. When I arrived, this young woman, in her mid-thirties, was lying in bed and appeared chronically ill, she was so thin and tired. For a month the pain in her back and right hip and leg had been increasing. My examination seemed to suggest the problem was emanating from the pelvis and hip bones, but I told the patient we would need x-rays to determine the cause. All I could do that night was give her something for the pain.

The couple then confessed that they had just returned from Des Moines, Iowa, where a well-known chiropractic medical center had given the woman a complete work-up. "Here's their report and the x-rays they took," the husband said, handing me a thick folder.

I read about the misplacements of my patient's vertebra and the shortening of her right leg which led to the tipping of the pelvis and her severe pain. The report also described the chiropractic manipulations that would alleviate her symptoms. In the last paragraph, I noticed a comment advising that if the lump in the patient's right breast persisted she should see a doctor. On films marked up with lines showing the angles for adjustments, I could see that the pelvis bone and right femur were riddled with cancer.

That was a sad evening as I gave this family the mother's diagnosis. Fortunately, she had several years left after her surgery and the radiation to the metastasis in her bone. She responded well to hormone manipulation and was able to continue working at her job and caring for her two young children. Years later we diagnosed her daughter with breast cancer, but it was caught at a much earlier stage, treated more effectively, and now, two decades later, this woman is disease-free.

During my first twenty years of practice, the tools for diagnosing bowel and abdominal cancers were as limited as those for breast cancer. If a person had a change in bowel habits, blood in the stool, or abdominal pain, we could do gastrointestinal studies which included an upper G-I (observing swallowed barium with fluoroscopy) or a barium enema (pushing in barium through the rectum and taking x-rays). Sometimes we would perform a sigmoidoscopy, which was looking at the lower eight to twelve inches of the rectum. Some adults would want a work-up every several years just due to the fear of developing cancer. If there was cancer and we could diagnose it early and remove it, usually the patient was cured. But often the diagnosis was too late. A patient would come in with a bloated abdomen and when we sent him to surgery, cancer would be discovered throughout the abdominal area. The surgery then became an open-and-shut procedure—the patient's fate sealed.

About thirteen years ago my daughter, Marlis, noticed numbness in her left foot and a tingling in the toes and ball of that foot. A podiatrist shot cortisone into her foot and recommended special running shoes with inserts. But the numbness persisted. Soon she started feeling severe pain in her left thigh and lower back. Marlis' family doctor in Ohio suggested a neurologist give her an EMG (Electromyogram). That test indicated the problem was not originating from her back as had been suspected, but from her brain.

Marlis felt certain she had multiple sclerosis, but an MRI revealed a large mass on the external, right side of the brain that looked like a meningioma. But she had experienced no headaches, no double vision, no obvious symptoms of a brain tumor. The next twenty-four hours were tense as our family waited for the intravenous contrast MRI that would indicate whether the tumor was cancerous. "I spent those hours trying to come to grips with the fact that I may not be here to raise my kids," Marlis recalls.

With great relief, we learned that the tumor was benign. There was a chance, however, that it was attached to the superior sagittal sinus, and, if that was the case, the surgeon would have to leave some of it behind. We were also concerned by the tumor's size—nearly that of a baseball.

Marlis had her craniotomy performed at the Fort Wayne Neurological Center where she felt so at ease she fell asleep laughing. The anesthesiologist had been razzing the attending nurse about graduating from Bluffton High School, and when he asked Marlis what she thought, she said, "Better not ask me my opinion. I graduated from Norwell!"

The surgery only took two and a half hours, instead of the expected four, and since the tumor wasn't attached to the sinus, the entire meningioma was extracted. Marlis said that she tried to insist on thirty-nine staples over the incision, to match her age, but they would only put in thirty-eight. She likes to tell a story about how five months later those staples set off the security system at Cincinnati's airport. In a *Markle Times* article, she joked, "My horseshoe incision goes undetected, unless there's a strong wind."

As a child, Marlis always enjoyed going with me on house calls and tagging along to the hospital, so it didn't surprise me when several years ago she decided to become a nurse. She received her degree in 2013 and currently works on a hospital's psychiatric ward. Dealing with the threat of cancer helped her realize she needed to follow her dream and that mid-life was not too late to begin.

In her poem, "Evening Chimes," Markle poet Alfreda Mossburg eloquently expresses what our family felt after Marlis' tumor was safely removed: deep gratitude to God and recognition of life's fragility. The last stanza goes:

Out of my soul the shadows flew,
Out of my heart a new song grew;
Out of the mouth a wordless prayer
As the chimes disappeared on the evening air.

ACCIDENTS

When I read about the early settlers in Huntington and Wells Counties, I'm struck by the high incidence of accidental deaths: men crushed by trees they were clearing, a farmer drowned when his boat capsized, another injured while working at the bottom of a well, an adolescent crushed and drowned by a waterwheel, a child mortally scalded when she fell into a bucket of hot water. In more recent times, our community has also grieved over victims of fatal accidents, most frequently of auto accidents, but sometimes it's been the calamity of a child breaking through river ice or of a farmer gouged by a bull.

Since Markle is a rural community, I came expecting to treat a number of farming accidents. Farming, according to the U.S. Bureau of Labor statistics, is more dangerous than roofing and almost as perilous as driving a truck. I knew from firsthand experience how easily serious accidents can happen on a farm. When I was twelve years old, one of my jobs was to fork down bedding straw for our cows. One day I was in a hurry to play outside, so I hastily spread the straw and then threw down the pitchfork. Later that afternoon my four-year-old sister walked barefoot into the barn, looking for me. My dad heard Sally Jo's screams and pulled a thick fork prong from the bottom of her foot. Dad's teenage brother died from an infected farm injury to his leg, so my parents immediately drove Sally Jo to the doctor. Unfortunately, she was severely allergic to the tetanus antitoxin and started swelling and breaking out in hives. She had trouble breathing and might have died if my parents hadn't rushed her back to Dr. Flannigan for a treatment of epinephrine and cortisone.

Most farmers in the Markle area concentrated on raising grain, rather than livestock, so I treated fewer injuries caused by animals than I initially expected. We did have two incidents of a bull mauling a farmer, though, and one ended in the farmer's death. I treated bites by farm dogs, and once even doctored a leg severely chewed by a hog.

Naturally, I saw injuries caused from farm machinery. The sharp teeth on corn pickers and shredders are notorious for chewing off farmers' fingers and even their hands. Mary's grandfather lost part of his hand in a corn shredder, and the famous Chicago Cubs pitcher from Nyesville, Indiana—Mordecai "Three Finger" Brown—mangled his hand in a shredder when he was five years old. To be accurate, Mordecai's injury wasn't actually an accident—his brother dared him to stick his hand in the shredder and Mordecai was someone who could never turn down a challenge. Fortunately, the accident worked to his advantage because he was able to perfect an odd breaking pitch with that hand, a pitch Ty Cobb called the "most devastating" he ever faced.

When the shredder responsible for Mordecai's injury retired, it was put on display across from the Nyesville Courthouse. I was relieved when the dangerous corn pickers in our area began to retire. I saw fewer hand injuries as farm machinery companies improved the safeguards on their new products.

But even with safety precautions, odd accidents happen. One evening I was called out to a farm south of Markle where a farmer lay in the field, trapped under his tractor. I do not remember how the tractor had turned over on him, but his leg was pinned and it was suspected that he had a period of unconsciousness. His vital signs were normal and except for a headache and leg pain, he said he felt okay. The ambulance took him to the hospital where x-rays of his head and leg ruled out any fractures. We kept him overnight, but the next day he went home.

Six weeks later I was called back to his home. The farmer had been feeling weak for about a week and was now running a fever and seemed confused. I had forgotten about the earlier injury because he had appeared so well when he left the hospital. In fact, he had quickly returned to his normal activities. Perplexed as to the cause of his symptoms, I had him transferred to Lutheran Hospital where I asked several different specialists to see him. The neurologist felt the problem was from a brain injury. This was before the development of CAT scans and MRIs, so an arteriogram of the brain was performed which indicated a large mass—a subdural hematoma. After his accident, bleeding between the brain and its coverings had caused pressure to slowly build. In order to drain the blood, a neurosurgeon drilled several burr holes in my patient's skull. Fortunately, this subdural hematoma was recognized in time—unlike the one I observed during my first year of medical school. During a routine examination, a group of my classmates found a large hematoma in the brain of their cadaver—the undiagnosed cause of that man's death.

With larger farm machinery and grain storage bins, I saw new types of injuries. One Rockcreek Township farmer suffocated in his grain bin before he could be reached. Another farmer, a close friend of mine, fell over thirty feet from the top of his grain bin and landed on cement. He stayed in Lutheran Hospital for many weeks with multiple fractures of his back, pelvis, and legs. However, with good emergency and specialized hospital care, he survived.

Not all of my patients were farmers. A number were factory workers who commuted to worksites in Fort Wayne, Huntington, or Bluffton. Others were employed locally by a company that coiled wires for generators—Square D—and by Wayne Metal Products. Before Wayne Metal built a larger, safer factory at the edge of town, I treated a lot of backs injured from lifting and fingers crushed or chopped off from the dangerous stamping machines. When a maker of prefabricated housing expanded in Markle, we started seeing more injuries to the hands and feet. I drilled holes in many fingernails to let blood out after hammer injuries. With nail guns it was difficult to pull a long nail out when it pierced clear through the shoe and foot.

It impressed me how these injured workers could withstand pain without complaint. It impressed Mary, too. One day while she was working the front desk at the office, a young man came up to the window asking to see the doctor. Mary said that he would have to wait about an hour until the doctors were back from lunch. "That's going to be hard for me to do," he said, calmly. "I have a nail through my foot."

Since the Markle area has a river, reservoir, quarry, creeks, ponds, and lakes, the potential for accidents involving water is always present. I felt the more swimming classes our young people could take the safer they would be so I was disappointed when, five years after our arrival, a campaign to add a swimming pool to the new Northern

Wells (Norwell) high school was defeated by those who felt it would be too expensive.

In the late 70s when the district was building a new middle school at the site of the high school, the chant rose again: "A Pool in the School." I was on the schoolboard then and heard the misgivings of other board members who felt there would be considerable opposition in the community over the extra expense. But the new drive for a pool was strengthened by the fact that in the preceding years there had been several drownings in area ponds and lakes. During the same summer that building plans were first being discussed, a recent Bluffton High School graduate—a tall, athletic boy, with a university scholarship from basketball—drowned in a local lake. He hadn't known how to swim.

The schoolboard called a public meeting about the issue of the pool and, expecting a huge turn-out, reserved the high school's auditorium. Thirty people came. Several rose to briefly say they supported the pool and the schoolboard's desire to make proficiency in swimming a requirement for students graduating from the eighth grade. After ten minutes a farmer stood up who said, "I can see I'm the only person against the pool. I guess it's time to go ahead and build it. Let's close the meeting and go home to watch IU play basketball."

That made sense, so we promptly disbanded. I don't remember who won the basketball game, but community safety scored a big win.

DRUG ABUSE

One Sunday afternoon I was watching the baseball game of the week when a mother called, disturbed about the condition of her teenage son.

"I don't know what's happened, but my son is acting scared," she said. "He says that his heart is going to jump out of his body, and he's seeing things that aren't there."

When I arrived, her son was clearly agitated and restless as he paced the living room floor. He had a tremor and scanning speech—speech in which syllables of words are separated by noticeable pauses. Although he seemed to recognize me and was cooperative, his statements were incoherent. He looked frightened, with dilated pupils and a rapid pulse. The boy's parents said they had noticed him this way for about an hour and that his condition was getting worse.

They also said that the mother of their son's friend called just before I arrived, saying her son was acting in a similar fashion, except she was having trouble keeping him from jumping out of his second-floor bedroom window. None of the parents had a notion as to what the boys might have taken. At the hospital I ordered blood tests and gave each boy a sedative. In a few hours their pulses had slackened and though they still acted frightened, one boy was rational enough to provide me with a clue—a newspaper clipping he withdrew from his pocket.

It reported that young people in California were being hospitalized from jimsonweed poisoning. These teens collected the spiky pods and then drank the crushed black seeds in their cokes. The ingestion of this weed, the article said, caused blurred vision, dilated pupils, elevated blood pressure, rapid pulse, dizziness, hallucinations, delirium, and possibly a coma and death. The boys told me they had crushed some jimsonweed seeds and tried them in their cokes. I asked if they hadn't read how this could kill them.

"We thought that was there to scare us," one boy replied. "They said that to keep us from trying the same thing, but we didn't think it was true."

After twenty-four hours of hospitalization, the boys were discharged. At the follow-up visit in the office, they told me that their experience with jimsonweed was so terrible that they'd never experiment with any drugs again.

When I told Shari about what had happened to the boys, it made such an impression on her that she decided to research the weed for her seventh grade science fair project. She discovered that jimsonweed, sometimes called *stinkweed, moonflower,* or *locoweed,* belongs to the nightshade family and that all parts are poisonous. Indigenous people throughout the world smoked or used a tea from this plant in supervised religious ceremonies or for medicinal purposes. The Zuni, for instance, used it as an anesthesia during the setting of broken bones and the Chinese during surgery. But the same tropane alkaloids that can provide medicinal benefit are fatally toxic in only a slightly larger dosage. Shari recognized the plant's stout stem, toothed leaves, and creamy, trumpet-shaped flowers near our creek, and as I drove to house calls, I began seeing jimsonweed all over Wells and Huntington counties, in roadside ditches and fields.

Though the lovely plant that Georgia O'Keefe painted in *Miracle Flower* is easy to procure, its effects are not easy to handle. Dr.Richard MacKenzie has aptly described its users as: "Hot as a hare, blind as a bat, dry as a bone, red as a beet, mad as a hatter." The ingestion or smoking of it for hallucinogenic effects isn't likely to ever become a serious trend since users seldom try it more than once.

Early in my practice I saw some patients who were addicted to the amphetamines in diet pills. Like the popular tapeworm tablets of the nineteenth and early twentieth centuries, these pills were effective in suppressing the appetite but had serious side effects. Patients addicted to the euphoric properties of amphetamines often experienced insomnia, restlessness, tremors, hallucinations, and behavioral changes. As I weaned people off of these pills, I tried to convince them that eating nutritious meals and getting regular exercise was a much healthier and sustainable means of weight control.

It wasn't until the last decade of my practice that the Markle Medical Center started seeing patients hooked to prescription painkillers like Oxycontin or Demerol. These patients weren't long-term residents of Markle, but people who traveled around a lot. They'd ask for a refill of their pain medication, but without really knowing their medical history, we had a difficult time determining whether the medicine was treating a legitimate pain or being procured to feed an addiction or to sell illegally. We soon made it a practice not to refill these prescriptions but to explore, instead, other treatment options such as anti-depressants or therapy at a rehabilitation center.

It is especially risky when a doctor becomes addicted to a narcotic because he or she has such easy access to refills. One of my friends, a doctor in another small town, started giving himself Demerol at night for gall bladder pains. After he finally had surgery, he took the drug for the post-surgery pain. Then he continued taking it because he had trouble handling the stress of his practice and Demerol helped him to sleep better.

One night he accidently shot the drug into an artery instead of a vein. When Demerol goes into a vein, it travels to the heart and is dispersed throughout the whole body; but when it's injected into an artery, it shoots straight down to the fingers, where it's so concentrated it will plug up the blood flow through the very small arteriolar and send them into spasms. If my friend hadn't gone to the hospital, he would have lost his fingers.

After that harrowing experience, my friend recognized his problem and asked me for help. I checked him into a rehab center in Minnesota, and he successfully stayed off of Demerol for the rest of his life.

As the result of an explosion, a methamphetamine lab was discovered in Markle on New Year's Day, 2014. The apartment was a "one-pot" lab, with a single soda bottle for mixing the chemicals. This was the first meth lab ever found in Markle, but such labs are a serious problem throughout Indiana, especially in rural areas and small towns. In 2013 Indiana ranked first in the country in the number of meth labs seized: one-thousand-eight-hundred-and-eight labs—eighty-two more than in the previous year.

Meth use may become a serious problem for the Markle area, but over the years, alcohol has been the drug most abused. The Markle Methodist Church used to devote one Sunday morning each year to the dangers of alcohol abuse. Elsie May Cline McGuffey, born in 1874, was always the speaker. Though Elsie died the year before I came to Markle, she is still remembered for dedicating considerable energy to the local Women's Temperance League.

As in many small-town communities, families usually kept alcohol problems hidden and dealt with them by trying their best to ignore them. Once I was called to a Markle home by the wife of a man who was shaking all over, sweating, and incontinent of urine, typical symptoms of alcohol withdrawal. He had the stomach flu (gastroenteritis) so I suspected that he was shaking because he couldn't keep down any alcohol. When I shared my suspicion with his wife, she said, "Oh, no, it can't be from that because he promised me he wouldn't drink anymore. He never goes to the tavern. He gave that up months ago." I told her to look for alcohol in the basement, behind boxes, in the garage, in any out of the way spaces. She called me later that day, saying she found bottles all over the property, some in quite obvious locations.

I had one patient who I first saw because her abdomen kept enlarging. She told me that she didn't drink alcohol, so I kept looking for other causes of liver failure. Finally, she admitted she was a closet alcoholic, addicted for over twenty years. She kept her secret by never drinking in public and never to excess.

One gentleman in Markle had so much fluid in his abdomen from liver failure that he would sew panels in the lower section of his shirts so he could close the buttons. To make him more comfortable, I tapped his abdomen on several occasions to drain fluid, but that also removed a considerable amount of proteins. His arms and legs were thin with muscle atrophy because of his poor nutrition and protein loss.

Whenever I suspected alcohol abuse, I encouraged patients to take a laboratory test so they would know if their liver was sensitive to alcohol and I could council them early before there was irreversible damage. But some patients I never saw for a drinking problem until it was too late.

Abraham Lincoln, who grew up in Spencer County, Indiana, once wrote, "The demon of intemperance ever seems to have delighted in sucking the blood of genius and of generosity. What one of us but can call to mind some relative more promising in youth than all his fellows, who has fallen a sacrifice to his rapacity?"

More often than not, some of the nicest people in the Markle community were the closet alcoholics.

THE BLUES

It was past midnight when the phone jarred me from sleep. A patient was anxious about her husband. They had argued bitterly that night, and he had stormed out. Now he wouldn't answer his office phone, and she was concerned he might hurt himself. "Please go to his office and see if he's okay," she pleaded. "The door will be unlocked if he's there."

I had helped this couple through some routine illnesses and marital conflicts. They were frequently separated so I wasn't surprised to learn that for the past several weeks the husband had been sleeping at his office.

His workplace was well-lit by an outdoor security light, but, inside, it was so dark I felt blindfolded. I called a name, but the only response was fierce barking. What was I doing there? Why hadn't I asked the town marshal to come along? As my eyes adjusted to the darkness, I saw a faint line of light beneath an interior door. I cautiously advanced, and on my way caught sight of two large, growling canines, each straining a chain that didn't quite reach me.

There was no response to my knock. Opening the door, I discovered that the light emanated from a small desk lamp. The man I had been looking for was slumped forward in his chair, with his arms across the desk and in one hand a gun. He didn't look up to acknowledge my presence, only kept staring at the pistol. His expression was tense. I noticed a large, uncapped bottle of scotch.

I greeted him and explained that his wife had called me because she loved him and was worried. He gave no response, just kept his gaze on the gun. I sat down on the

134

nearby couch and started telling him that I knew how badly he felt and described what I thought he might be feeling— anger and hopelessness. I explained that with some help, he could feel much better. He still did not respond, so I just kept talking. I said how I admired the way he had developed a successful business and could keep it running in such hard economic times. I talked as the wall clock ticked. Suddenly, he started sobbing. He put down the gun and began talking about what was depressing him—marital problems, conflicts with his children, and business difficulties.

About an hour and a half later, he emptied the bullets and poured the liquor down the drain. He promised to sleep and then see me in the office that afternoon. I planned to start him on an antidepressant and arrange counseling for him and his wife.

This was not the kind of house call I ever expected to encounter when I envisioned myself practicing medicine in a rural area. I seldom even heard the word "depression" as I was growing up. In the Shipshewana community, as in many other places in the United States, depression was a family secret. The only person I knew who was described as depressed was one of my aunts who I remember frequently crying. I never knew of anyone in our Mennonite church of two hundred members who suffered depression, though surely there were those who did. In his essay, "Scatter Plots: Depression, Silence, and Mennonite Margins," Jeff Gundy claims that the tendency of Swiss Mennonites to be patient and emotionally reticent has often caused depression in their communities to go unrecognized. He writes, "We tend to assume that because we do care for each other, we don't need to talk about it much, and that things are generally all right as long as we can't find much to say about them. Mostly this serves us well, but if things are not all right, we have little practice at the kind of discourse that we need."

As Gundy later acknowledges, Mennonites don't have a corner on reticence. During my practice, especially in the early years, I found people in Markle and the surrounding rural community also reserved when it came to talking about their grief or doubts or losses. There was a strong sense of fortitude and self-sufficiency that, on one hand, I admired but, on the other, made my diagnosis of depression more difficult.

When I finished medical school, I was much better prepared to deal with hypertension and peptic ulcer disease than depression. It was only covered briefly in psychiatry courses, and there was no discussion of outpatient treatment or how to provide counseling. My class did tour Logansport Mental Hospital where we observed depressed people in an institutional setting, sitting in large, dreary rooms, looking dejected. We watched patients getting electroshock and insulin shock therapy. We even saw some receiving hydrotherapy, a treatment in which they were immersed alternately from ice cold to intensely hot baths.

A few weeks before I moved to Markle, a doctor who had previously worked in that area asked if I wanted to make a house call with him to see a child in Markle who had the flu. I jumped at the opportunity to see an experienced doctor at work in a community where I would soon be practicing, but what I remember most about our trip that day was him pointing out houses where someone had committed suicide. House after house, there were so many that the trip left me unnerved.

Fortunately, antidepressants were on the market soon after I started my practice. I would rate their development as similar to the breakthrough in the discovery of penicillin. But in addition to dispensing medication, I knew it was important to build a strong rapport with my depressed patients so they would feel comfortable calling me day or night, whenever they felt in a hopeless situation. On one house call, I met with a man in a barn who was thinking about hanging himself from a rafter. Another time, I spoke through the door to a woman who had locked herself in her bedroom. In the 60s, people did not want to hear the word *depression* so I had a lot of teaching to do and often used synonyms such as *sadness, the dumps,* or *the blues.*

Over the course of my practice no one committed suicide whom I had diagnosed as depressed. However, some people took their lives who I didn't know were depressed because they hadn't come to the office or they came with another unrelated ailment and I was not sharp enough to sense their despondency. Over the years, though, I became more alert to recognizing the underlying depression that is often a part of a related illness.

The water tower in Markle has a smiley face painted on the tank, but instead of yellow, its color is blue. It reminds me that any life has its joys and its sorrows and that the sadness should not be hidden or denied.

NEAR-DEATH EXPERIENCES

During my third year in medical school, I worked a morning rotation at the Veterans Hospital in Indianapolis. Each day my group—a resident, intern, senior medical student, and I—started out by making rounds to all the patients on our floor. Sometimes a staff physician accompanied us. One morning we were on our tenth-floor rounds when a nurse hollered, "Visitor down in the hall!" We ran a few yards to a man sprawled across the floor. He wasn't breathing. He had no pulse and was turning blue.

The resident took charge and had us place our patient in a bed with a board underneath him. Then we started external chest compressions and mouth to mouth breathing until we could get an endotracheal tube down his throat and hook him to oxygen. We started IV fluids and took an EKG reading. He was in ventricular fibrillation so we gave him an electroshock—and then several more, each with increasing power. Finally, his sixty-five-year-old heart started beating on its own and his blood pressure returned. I wondered if this man would have brain damage, but the next morning he was propped up in bed reading the newspaper. He said he was fine except that his chest was sore—especially when he coughed.

In 1962 the successful closed resuscitation of a sudden cardiac arrest was a reportable event, and the resident and staff physician wrote up this incident in a medical journal. Before this time, most successful attempts involved open heart massage and defibrillation.

During our first year of practice, Lee and I performed a similar resuscitation. After diagnosing a sixty-three-year-old Markle businessman with bowel cancer, we admitted him to Lutheran Hospital and referred him to a surgeon. On the patient's fifth post-operative day, Lee and I were making rounds together when we walked into the patient's private room and observed him taking what seemed like his last breath: he had no pulse and was turning blue. We pressed the patient's nurse call button and started CPR. Soon nurses came running to help and bring what we needed. This was long before hospitals had code blues, IV teams, or organized resuscitation teams. Though it took some time to bring a defibrillator to the room, we, nevertheless, had a successful resuscitation. This patient was cured of his cancer and lived a number of healthy years after his near-death experience.

On November 21, 1980, my patient, James Fuller, had an experience that still amazes me. That Friday morning, having finished my rounds, I stopped by the Wells Community Hospital's new coronary care unit to watch Jim perform a treadmill test. He had been experiencing some tightness in his chest and pain in his arm, neck, and jaws. Jim had first complained to his wife, Pat, the previous week when his chest burned as if he had been "running very fast in cool air."

Jim was our nearby neighbor and worked at the International Harvester Company in Fort Wayne, operating machines that made gears for truck transmissions. He was forty seven years old and had always been in good health. His three children—Vickie, Amy, and Tracy—were good friends with my children and in the same grades. As Jim took the treadmill test, Lee, who was monitoring it, noted that his

EKG and cardiac functions seemed to be normal. But after the nurses removed the electrodes and Jim began pulling on his t-shirt, an intense pain seized him. He told the nurses, "You're going to have to let me lie down because something is happening."

A few weeks after his heart attack, Jim wrote about what happened. Here is his remarkable story:

As I was lying down, someone raised my tongue and put some tablets under it. (I found out later they were nitroglycerin pills.) At the same time, oxygen tubes were put in my nose and someone was pulling off my shoes and clothes. By this time, the pain was so intense that it felt as if a tremendous pressure was trying to separate my head from my neck—right at my jaws. In fact, my jaws hurt so badly I felt no pain anywhere else. Only half conscious, I remember answering the nurses or doctors, but I don't really know what I said. I think I may have passed out for a few seconds, and I thought I was given a shot in the thigh. I know I was semi-conscious when they put me on a cart and wheeled me into Coronary Care. The pain was much less by now. As I passed under the lights in the hall, I thought, 'Is this the last thing I will see in this life?' Yet I had no fear or feeling that I was going to die.

I was aware of being lifted off the cart into a bed in the CC Unit and of doctors and nurses around me, doing something. At this time, I had no pain. But then a strange thing happened. A total silence filled the room and my spirit left my body. I seemed (or rather, my spirit seemed) to be whole—I mean, with feet, arms, legs and everything. Yes, and even dressed. But my spirit was floating above and to the right of the body in the bed. At that time, I was not interested in the body lying in the bed or the people around it, because a hole with a bright light at the other side appeared in the wall. The light was very bright, but it didn't hurt my eyes; it seemed to draw me towards it. I had the feeling of complete peace, unlike any feeling in life, and I wanted to go through that hole in the wall. I moved toward it, but when I got there, the hole moved off to my left. Instantly, without any feeling of movement, I was—or my spirit was—perched back where it had been.

All was the same in the room: the body in bed, people standing around it, but the hole in the wall had moved. I tried once more to go to that hole in the wall, but I felt a hand on my shoulder, restraining me. I don't know why I didn't look to see who it was, but I didn't. At the time it just seemed natural for this event to take place. There were no spoken words, but there registered in my mind a message from the person whose hand was on my shoulder. The message was: 'It is not your time.' Those may have not been the exact words, but that was their meaning.

The hole still appeared in the wall, moving first one place, then another, but I didn't try to go through. I just sat, perched there, watching what was going on below. I guess I knew then that the body on the bed below was going to live. One of the persons put something against my chest and, instantly, the spirit and body were together and my body seemed to jump rather violently, still with no pain or feeling. Just as instantly, the spirit was back up on his perch observing. I was told later that the jumping was the reaction of my body to the electric shock that was being used to start my heart. This same event—the jerking and the spirit entering and leaving the body—happened, what seemed to me, three times. I then heard the voice of Dr. Lee Kinzer. Prior to that, I (my spirit) could not even distinguish the doctors from the nurses around the body; they were just figures—people. Dr. Kinzer said, "Jim, we are going to insert a pacemaker and this might hurt a little." Instantly, my spirit was back in my body. I felt no more

141

than a pin-prick, and then I went to sleep, not to awaken until eight that night.

Jim told us exactly what we had been doing during the procedure, even when he had been without blood pressure. He knew who had held the defibrillator and where each of us stood. His eyes had been closed during that whole time, except when we opened his eyelids to see if his pupils remained constricted.

In reflecting upon his near-death experience, Jim wrote:

One thing I would like to bring out was that while in the spirit, I had no concept of time. I thought it was hours, when, in reality, Dr. Kinzer told me that it was only about 20 to 30 minutes from the time the attack started until the pacemaker was inserted. Also, when in my spirit form, I could float right through the figures around the body on the bed. Another thing was, after it was over, I felt a little guilty about the fact that, while in spirit form, I had no feeling at all for my body and not once did my spirit think of my wife, my family and my loved ones. I guess that is the way of death—I don't know.

From this experience, I have learned that material things don't really mean that much. Life means more than hard work. . . Enjoy what you already have because, when the time comes, you won't take anything with you, not even your body, through that hole.

Pat said that after this experience Jim was different. He had no fear of dying, and he didn't worry as much or get irritated when things went wrong. When he thought about dying, his only regret was that he wouldn't see his grandson grow up.

Jim had coronary bypass surgery about three weeks after Lee inserted a pacemaker. Eight years later, his heart problems started to return and during his second surgery he died from a blood clot. "That time," Pat told me, "Jim went through the light and stayed."

I have read about other near-death experiences—many of them with details about moving through a tunnel, gazing down at one's own body, meeting again with deceased loved ones, and being overwhelmed with a feeling of peace—but the cases that have been most meaningful to me are the ones that have happened to my own patients. One older gentleman was in church when he collapsed. Because the Methodist Church was across from the ambulance service and a doctor from our group was in the congregation, as well as a couple of nurses, resuscitation efforts began immediately and were successful. This man later said, "I felt myself leave my body, and then I was lifted up toward a bright light with what I felt were angels lining the way. It was comforting, and I was not scared."

A few years later, one of my patients experienced something less comforting. This time the patient was a woman in her fifties, with two children. She had pancreatic cancer and was losing weight. She had a rough life, with many bad habits, and she expressed no spiritual leanings. One afternoon she started hemorrhaging from her stomach. Immediately, she became faint and anxious. Her husband helped her into the car and started driving to the hospital, fifteen miles away. "Go faster, go faster. This is terrible! Go faster," the woman screamed. Before her husband reached the hospital, she was unconscious. In the emergency room, the team started fluids, oxygen, and vasopressors to raise her blood pressure and gave her blood transfusions.

When my patient regained consciousness, she was still agitated. She told me that on the way to the hospital her spirit left her body. "I felt myself going down a long, dark staircase where I couldn't see the bottom," she said. "Scary things were all around me—like I was going to hell."

Her life underwent a spiritual transformation after this event—as did the lives of her husband and a daughter. She sought reconciliation with others, and when, six months later, her husband again rushed her to the hospital, he related that she was at peace. As she lost consciousness in the car, she said, "I love you. Don't be afraid. I'm dying, but it's okay."

When it comes to my faith in God and in an afterlife, I find that what I learn from science only strengthens my faith by making me feel more keenly the wonder and mystery that sustains our every breath. One of my favorite Hoosier writers, the naturalist and novelist Gene Stratton-Porter, looked closely at the world and found her faith confirmed by what she observed. "In the economy of nature nothing is ever lost," she wrote. "I cannot believe that the soul of man shall prove the one exception."

FOUR: A PLACE IN THE PARADE

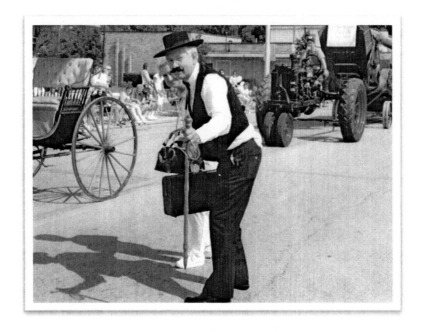

AN HONORARY GROUCH

One of the best things about being a rural, small-town doctor is how well you get to know your patients. You see them at the grocery store, ballgames, restaurants, and in church. You sit next to them in the dentist's waiting room and pump gas at the same station. Some professionals do not like interacting with clients outside their workplace, but I enjoyed it and did not even mind being asked medical questions. Just as patients asked for my advice, I asked for theirs. For instance, not being mechanically minded or knowledgeable in carpentry or plumbing, I'd often seek my patients' assistance on what I should do or whom I should contact when there was a problem with my car or house.

As our practice expanded, with patients coming from as far as thirty miles away, Lee and I also appreciated how community people looked out for us by trying to protect our privacy. One of Lee's favorite stories involved Mary Randol who worked at Hoover's Hardware. One time Lee's brother on leave from mission work in East Africa walked into the hardware store to ask directions to Dr. Kinzer's house.

Assuming this man was a patient, Mary said, "Dr. Kinzer is awful busy. He works too many hours. I can't tell you where he lives."

Lee's brother responded, "But I came all the way from Africa to see him!"

The people of Markle were more than our patients. They were neighbors and friends whom we enjoyed helping out and learned to know better through community organizations and activities.

The first organization Lee and I joined was the Lions Club. Our annual fundraiser was for an eye bank, and to collect money, we'd walk door to door, selling light bulbs and brooms. We also gathered the signatures of people willing to donate their corneas to the Indiana University Eye Center. Though our local chapter closed in the late 70s, for years afterward I was still going to area funeral homes to extract the eyes of those who had made donations.

The Lion's Club, Psi Iota Xi, and a few other organizations teamed up to plan the Halloween party each year. On All Hallows' Eve, Morse Street smelled of sloppy joes and was blocked off so children dressed as hobos, witches, or monsters with humped shoulders could rush freely from vendor to vendor. They bobbed for apples or cast lines hooked with safety pins over a sheet to fish for trinkets. Blindfolded, they crawled through a haunted house where peeled grapes and soft pasta suggested anatomical horrors.

Adults often dressed up, too. I was stalked my first year by a full-sized mummy who kept asking me to guess who he was. I had no idea since I was a newcomer and couldn't recognize the voice. Most adults congregated near the cake walk or waited in line to take aim at a lever that sent members of the Lions Club plummeting into six feet of water. I can attest to the fact that Halloween nights back then were always chilly—as was the water in the dunking tank. Like the other men who took the "hot seat," I urged on customers by taunting, "Hey, you couldn't hit me if you were three feet away" or "Come on, come on, let's see you wind up your arm." Perched four feet above the water, we dared our own downfall.

I also helped with Markle Progress Day, an event sponsored by the town's Business Association and held on the Saturday of Labor Day weekend. A morning bicycle parade crossed over the bridge to the park where townspeople converged. The day featured helium balloons tied to children's wrists, barbecued chicken, gunny sack and three-legged races, and an afternoon softball game between the Sod Busters and City Slickers. In the evening the capstone event was a talent show with barbershop quartets, skits, baton twirling, and instrumentals. One year a man stacked nails—dozens of nails balanced on top of each other. Another year our good friend, Jean Mossburg, brandished a long cigarette holder as she spoke despairingly of her husband, Fang, and cackled at her own jokes. Her first place performance as Phyllis Diller revealed that Jean might have had a comedic stage career if she had left her hometown.

During my turn as president of the Markle Business Association, we decided that posting signs would be a good way to welcome visitors and encourage them to slow down. There were five major entrances into town so we chose five "Welcome to Markle" slogans: "Slow down, you may want to stop." "Slow down, we love our children." "If you lived here, you would be home now." "A town with a history and a future." The fifth sign was by far the most original: "Welcome to Markle, a town of 910 happy people and 3 grouches." This sign sparked considerable interest, and people speculated as to the identity of the grouches. Three doctors now worked at the medical center and some suggested they might be the malcontents.

In 1981, thirteen years later, the population of Markle had increased and so had the number of town grouches—to four. That was the year Mary, as a member of the planning committee for the Markle Wildcat Festival (an event that replaced Progress Day), conceived of an annual grouch contest as a way to heighten festival interest. "Why don't we have a contest to name our four grouches?" she asked the committee. She received some strange looks but was unanimously elected to chair the Grouch Committee. For a quarter a vote you could help elect your favorite good-natured grouch who lived or worked in Markle. Coffee cans with slits for ballots and coins were placed at area businesses, and the four nominees with the highest ballot count would serve as honorary town grouches for one year.

That first contest was a huge success though Mary says to some extent it backfired since she was elected one of the grouches. So were two of the other committee members— Jean Mossburg and the local mortician, Bruce Myers. Along with Lavone Miller, the drugstore clerk, they all received a plaque commemorating their election and rode the lead convertible in the Princess Wildcat Parade. The committee was concerned how Lavone would react to being elected a grouch, but she responded with grace. During the parade she said, "This is sure fun," and, "I'm going to live up to my title."

The election of town grouches has continued to become a beloved Markle tradition that has helped put the town on the map. Ripley's *Believe It or Not* included a description in one of its editions, and in 1983 a reporter for the *Indianapolis Star* wrote: "If its advertising can be trusted, the northeast Indiana town of Markle must be a great place to live. After all, it would seem an easy task to avoid a mere four grouches among a population of more than 900. Unfortunately, Markle's grouches change every year."

Mary helped with the grouch contest for twenty-three years and tried to emphasize during each election period that it was a *positive* distinction to be voted a town grouch — and in *no way* an indication that you really *were* a grouch. She only remembers one year when an elected grouch declined the position, saying he had a fishing trip to Michigan planned. If rumor was right, he had nothing scheduled but skipped town to avoid the recognition. Having been an honorary grouch myself, I concur with Mary that the distinction is purely an indication of popularity and a tribute of public esteem.

Initially, I had the Welcome to Markle signs cut from plywood and hired a local painter to add the lettering. When these signs grew weathered, metal ones replaced them. Now all five entrances carry an attractive, updated version of only the favorite greeting. It indicates that the happy population has grown to 1,102, whereas the grouch count has stabilized at four.

THE MARKLE WILDCAT FESTIVAL

In the Bicentennial year of 1976 the Markle Business and Community Association decided to change the name of Markle Progress Day in order to pay homage to the Miami who once had a village nearby. The celebration's new name specifically honored Chief *Peshewa* ("The Wildcat") and his wife *Natoequah* who had once owned land along Markle's southern riverfront.

Not much is known about Natoequah, whose name also appears as *Wapenquah* on a local land grant, but Peshewa, whose French name was Jean Baptiste de Richardville, was the son of a French fur-trader and his mother was *Tacumwa*, an influential Miami political leader and businesswoman. Peshewa's uncles included the famous war chief Little Turtle and the hereditary chief *Pacanne*.

Peshewa owned a brick, two-story home in *Kikionga* (Fort Wayne) that is now a national historic landmark, but what is not well known is that he also had a more traditional home in the Miami village near Markle. An early settler in Huntington County, William Coolman, once found refuge on what was called the Wildcat or Richardville Reserve—within Peshewa's own cabin. While trying to locate his plat of land near what is now Warren, this pioneer from Gettysburg, Ohio lost his way in the snow and was nearly freezing to death when he heard dogs barking and children hollering. Markle historian Milfort Lambert writes in a *Markle Times* article that the sounds drew him to Peshewa's cabin where "the Miami treated the wandering, lost man with great kindness."

Peshewa and his mother amassed great wealth from operating a portage between the St. Mary's and Wabash Rivers, part of a pathway connecting commerce between Canada and the Gulf of Mexico. At his death in 1841 legend claims Peshewa was the wealthiest Native American in the United States due to the tolls from this portage and individual land grants from the federal government. But historian Stewart Rafert writes that at Peshewa's death there was no evidence he left great wealth: "Hereditary chiefs among the Miami were expected to be generous to their people, and Richardville fulfilled this role. Aiding the distressed in the tribe was the key to his leadership status."

The treaties that Peshewa helped negotiate delayed the Miami Removal until 1846, five years after his death, and succeeded in allowing half of the tribe to remain in Indiana after the Removal. General John Tipton described Peshewa's influence in a letter to Secretary of War John Eaton in 1831: "The Miamis are reduced to a small number—but well organized in their kind of government, and with one of the most shrewd men in North America at their head."

In 1838 Peshewa affixed only an "X" to the land agreement for Wildcat Reserve, a grant co-signed by President Tyler. But that X does not signify that he could not write his name. As a young man Peshewa received schooling in Quebec and became fluent in three languages—Miami, French, and English. His refusal to sign his name was part of his ideological resistance to European and American culture. After the Treaty of St. Mary's in 1818, a treaty Peshewa felt was unjust, he shunned what he had earlier adapted— French and American clothing, music, and language.

If they were alive today, Peshewa and Natoequah might shun the same festival that's named in their honor, but I think they would appreciate that this event brings Markle people together for a day of strengthening communal ties. They might also appreciate the competitive nature of the games. A cultural trait of the Miami is their love of games; in fact, shooting matches were popular between the Miami and Markle's first settlers.

From the festival's inception, Mary was an active member of the planning committee, frequently serving as chairperson or assistant chair. As treasurer of the Markle Business and Community Association and later on, the Chamber of Commerce, she naturally wanted the event to be a success, but she also truly took pleasure in the creative and social aspects of organizing a full weekend of community entertainment.

My wife was perennially on the lookout for unique activities to add to the Festival's traditional list of events that included the Princess Wildcat Pageant, the Saturday morning parade, the Grouch Contest, Tennis Tourney, Firemen's Water Battle, and Sunday's Classic Car Show. Over the years she introduced such new activities as camel and helicopter rides, a threshing demonstration, an 1875 chuck wagon and encampment, and a squirrel photo contest.

One year, when Mary was chairperson, her phone rang and she couldn't believe who was on the line—a circus manager. He said his circus would be passing through on State Route 224 and he wondered if it could take part in the Wildcat Festival. She felt obliged to explain that Markle was a small town and there wasn't much room in the park for a circus, but that didn't bother him. He said that the circus wouldn't be much trouble for the town; all it had to do was to publicize the event and sell the five dollar tickets. Mary said she'd need to check with the planning committee and then she'd call back.

Not wanting to take a chance that the circus manager might change his mind, she hurried downtown to see who she could find from the committee. Bill Randol who was in his insurance office thought a circus show would be a wonderful event and even volunteered to take charge.

Late that summer, on a Friday afternoon, the crowd watched as elephants helped raise the big tent. The same elephants promenaded in next morning's parade and gave afternoon rides. The Franzen Circus presented two big top shows on Saturday, and people packed the stands to watch performing lions, horses, acrobats, and clowns.

Another year Mary heard about an outhouse race that the town of Warren had sponsored for Salamonie Days. Fort Wayne and some other local communities held hospital bed races, but Mary thought an outhouse race sounded more challenging and might bring back memories from the past. Older Markle residents could remember when each home had an outhouse; in fact, a few houses still kept a dilapidated one in the backyard.

Mary borrowed two plain, single-seat outhouses from Warren. These privies had doors missing and skids with small rollers so they could be pushed. Eight Markle businesses agreed to compete in the race. The Markle Medical Center selected Dr. Dave Brown and me to be pushers and the lightest nurse on staff, Janet Himes, to be the rider perched upon the hole. The preliminaries would entail four races to reduce the field to four teams and then the semifinals would narrow those teams down to the final two.

With a surgical mask hanging from our neck and a layer of green surgical scrubs over our clothes, Dave and I looked professional as we took our places behind our outhouse. However, this was possibly the hottest day in Festival history and with the strip of blacktop between the softball diamond and the quarry radiating the sun's sweltering noonday heat, we were already sweating before the gun went off.

Dave and I won the first heat easily. During the preliminaries there was some extra excitement when one team lost control of their privy—it veered, skidding toward the fence where bystanders were at risk. Fortunately, the renegade outhouse was captured while still on the asphalt.

The semifinals were much harder since Dave and I were getting tired and increasingly hot. We won this time by only a foot. That brought us to the finals, to face the Nodine Dentistry team. Now, Dave and I were not in the best physical condition, but we made up for it by being the most competitive. With fans cheering, we pushed on—against weak legs, racing hearts, shirts wet with perspiration. We pushed to victory. Thereafter, we collapsed. I passed out for a few moments and when I awoke found myself surrounded by nurses and EMTs. It took a while to find my voice, but I remember telling them that I was okay, to just let me rest.

Accused of trying to finish me off, Mary never ordered any more privies from Warren. She made sure that her new events were safer, with less physical exertion. The Duck Race was a disaster because the plastic ducks that took off on the river got stuck in the reeds, but the moon pie eating competition, the squirrel photo contest, and the diaper derby went off without a hitch. Millie's Movement required some patience on the part of the crowd, but it, too, was a success. It was a little like bingo, and no undue exertion was needed, at least in the human sphere. The Mautz family brought Millie, their cow, to the park, where she grazed on a shady parcel of roped off grass, with squares marked and numbered. They would feed Millie a snack and then everyone watched to see on what square she made her deposit.

On second thought, Peshewa and Natoequah might relate best to the evening swing or line dances that are traditionally a part of The Wildcat Festival. The Miami used to hold large dances in a field adjacent to the confluence of the Wabash and the Rock Creek, in a field about a mile and a half south of town.

A few years ago, Jerry and Jean Mossburg took Mary, Shari, and me to this field. Jerry's great-great-grandfather, Daniel Mossburg, met his future wife, Elizabath Brown, while both were spectators here. That was in 1840: six years before the Removal; a year before Peshewa's death; one hundred and thirty-six years before the first Wildcat Festival.

Time flows forward like the Wildcat Parade—carrying along the past and the present. Now that field, once filled with drumbeat and song, is waist high in Queen Anne's lace and thistle. Interstate 69 passes nearby, but traffic is hidden by a remnant of forest and muffled by the sound of water over stone.

THE BOYS WHO CAME BEFORE

Though we scraped his name off the front window and poured his Rhubarb Elixir down the drain, Dr. Haldon Woods was someone I thought a lot about my first years in Markle. Naturally, he was mentioned as patients told me their histories. I learned that it wasn't uncommon for him to stop at a house for a cup of coffee and then check on a patient while there. One family—the Souers—told me they thought so highly of the doctor they named their son Haldon.

One woman remembered that when she started feeling labor pains, Doc Woods drove to her home that Sunday evening and timed the contractions while they watched *The Loretta Young Show*. As the episode ended he stood up and said, "It's time to go." The doctor followed his patient and her husband to the hospital and delivered the baby before midnight.

I learned a few things about Dr. Woods in *The Markle Times* that allowed me to see him outside of his professional role. For instance, he loved old cars—especially one model a patient had restored: a 1930 Chrysler Model 66, the same car Eliot Ness drove on the television show, *The Untouchables*. Haldon admired this car so much that the vehicle's owner let him drive it to a medical convention in Indianapolis.

When he wasn't treating patients, the doctor also liked to farm. He raised enough tomatoes to sell to a small local factory where the best ones were canned and the second-best made into ketchup. Given the amount of Elixir we found in his office, I have a hunch he also raised his own rhubarb.

It felt right to be carrying on a tradition of health care in which the physician was an integral part of the community. Eventually, I discovered that this tradition stretched back more than a century to include many Markle doctors.

In 1850 the town's first doctor settled in a village that only existed on paper. Fifteen years earlier the land had been platted, but trees still grew thick and nobody lived there. When Dr. Joseph Scott arrived, he would have seen the remains of a house a man with the surname of Tracy built in 1832. Mr. Tracy constructed this house by hand—down to splitting the shingles—and then went back East to fetch his family. But the years passed; the man never returned. No one ever lived in that house with black walnut shingles. According to legend, a tree took root and grew through the hole where the stone chimney would have stood.

Dr. Scott was twenty-six years old when he moved to Markle (then called Tracy). He grew up in Massillon, Ohio where he studied under an older doctor for four years before attending medical lectures in Cleveland. Young Doc Scott must have had an adventurous spirit. How else could he have survived in the wilderness, especially without a horse? After he built the first frame home on the north bank of the Wabash, he was too poor to afford even a mule and had to make his house calls on foot. That entailed a good deal of walking since his practice consisted entirely of house calls and the countryside was sparsely settled. Dr. Scott reportedly saved time by taking short-cuts through the forest, yet I suspect those short-cuts might also have been the source of his many "interesting as well as startling experiences" alluded to but never detailed in an 1887 history of Huntington County. Wolves, bears, cougars, and rattlers inhabited the forest, and as he hiked at night toward the home of an expectant mother or a farmer recovering from ague, his lantern might have illumined these.

Whether he walked under giant trees (some five feet in diameter) or along rough roads, the doctor would have traversed through mud, particularly in Huntington County's Rock Creek Township. Elizabeth Strouse told F.S. Bash that "it was mud, mud, mud—the stickiest, blackest mud that any mortal ever got into!" Only two and a half miles west of Markle was a spot known to sink wagon wheels up to their hubs. Dr. Scott must surely have skirted "Devil's Half Mile," where thieves hid in wait for mired travelers.

But I don't think thieves would have found much cash on Dr. Scott, at least in the early 1850s. Although the farmland surrounding Markle was fertile, money was scarce and the doctor was often paid with corn, pork, coonskins, or just a hearty meal. When the doctor married in January, 1852, he was "in very straitened circumstances." In fact, the doctor had to borrow money for the marriage license and to pay the justice of the peace.

Dr. Scott eventually bought a horse and his practice expanded to cover parts of three counties—southern Huntington and portions of Wells and Grant. By 1856 he wasn't the only doctor in Markle, but he retained a reputation as one of the region's most skilled and successful. He also gained repute as someone active in public affairs and a prominent member of the local Republican Party. Dr. Scott was an early township trustee and in 1857 was appointed Markle's postmaster, a job he held for ten years though his annual compensation was only three dollars. The doctor might have found it convenient to carry his post office with him—on top of his head. A few years earlier, Markle's first postmaster, Amos Curry, did that. He kept the mail "in his old ash colored plug hat," said Matilda Roush, who was a young girl then.

Dr. Scott was still living in Markle when he died at age sixty-five—twelve years younger than I am now. Before he died, he was described as an old man of good health and "strong physical endurance" but "broken somewhat from exposure." This leads me to think that the years without a horse and the decades of riding horseback to house calls in three counties may have aged him prematurely.

The next Markle doctor I know of is Henry L. Zumro. To my knowledge he is the only Markle physician to have worked as an undercover agent for the U.S. government. He's also the inspiration for Dr. Delphus Duall in Ulysses S. Lesh's novel, *A Knight of the Golden Circle.* Mr. Lesh, born near Markle in 1868, was a lawyer by trade. If his description of Dr. Duall accurately depicts Dr. Zumro, then the real doctor "was a small man with sharp black eyes—well matching his full black whiskers—and of such a penetrating character as to add almost irresistible force to his diplomatic tongue. He had been well schooled for his profession, and for several years had been the leading physician of the village and surrounding community."

Dr. Zumro had practiced medicine in Markle for ten years when he was recruited during the Civil War to infiltrate local chapters of the Order of the Sons of Liberty. This was another name for The Knights of the Golden Circle, an underground society that formed in the South, in 1854, with the goal of establishing a slave-holding empire with its capitol in Havana, Cuba. The radius of this "golden circle" would extend 1,200 miles to include St. Louis, Baltimore, Central America, and Mexico. The organizers hoped that President Buchanan would allow states to pull out of the union without resistance and that this new realm would then have a monopoly on cotton, rice, sugar, and tobacco.

During the Civil War, Northerners who strongly sympathized with the South formed secret chapters of The Knights of the Golden Circle in Ohio, Indiana, Illinois, and Iowa. These men were usually Peace Democrats, also called Copperheads, who fervently supported State's rights and feared that economic and governmental trends threatened their agrarian lifestyle. Dr. Zumro testified in court that when he joined The Sons of Liberty he was told the object of the organization was to "subdue the Abolitionists, resist the draft, and to assist the Southern Confederacy."

Through his undercover work, the doctor exposed a plot to free Confederate soldiers in an Indianapolis prison and arm them. In 1865 he testified in a military court against one of the designers of this plan—Lambdin Milligan, a Huntington attorney. Lambdin was found guilty of treason and scheduled to hang, but President Lincoln pigeon-holed the orders and later a Supreme Court review released him from prison, determining that he and the other leaders involved in the plot should have been tried in a civilian court of their peers, setting the legal precedent of *Ex parte Milligan*.

I don't know what happened to Dr. Zumro after the trial. Did he continue his practice in Markle? Or did some community resentment cause him to move on to another town or state? During the proceedings Milligan's attorney brought in witnesses from the Markle area who testified that the doctor's word was not to be trusted. However, the prosecution brought in an equal number of witnesses who said his word could be trusted. It took great courage to do what Dr. Zumro did. He would have known he was jeopardizing his practice, not to mention those friendships that crossed political lines. In court he explained that his purpose in joining the secret order "was not to betray its members, but to keep the Government posted as to their designs." "There appeared to be a great danger of an outbreak and rebellion at home," he explained, "and I thought if I could do anything to prevent it, I was doing the community a kindness, and not injury."

Dr. Henry C. Gemmill was perhaps the best educated of Markle's nineteenth-century physicians. He arrived in 1882 after reading medicine with two doctors in Logansport, Indiana and graduating from one of the nation's top medical schools—Rush Medical College in Chicago. Dr. Gemmill had lived in Markle for only four years before he was elected president of the Huntington County Medical Society.

The doctor's paternal grandfather was a Scottish sea captain and his parents were hardworking farmers who moved from Virginia to Cass County, Indiana when their son was thirteen. Four years later, young Gemmill enlisted in the Indiana infantry and was seriously wounded that same year at the Battle of Richmond, Kentucky. At that point, the Union soldier who would become one of Markle's most highly-regarded doctors was discharged and could have avoided any more battles. But when he recovered, he proceeded to enlist again and served as a sergeant until the war's end.

From talking with a patient who was almost ninety, I learned that in the 1920s Markle had seven doctors. I wish I had asked Verna Stockman for their names because she was still so sharp I think she could have recalled them. From the *History of Huntington County*, I do know the town's four doctors in 1914: Marvin F. Fisher, Robert G. Johnston, William J. Kilander, and Arthur H. Northrup. Dr. Kilander, however, was age seventy-six at the time, so his practice might have been fairly limited. Both he and Dr. Northrup are buried in Markle's cemetery, the latter near his daughter, Evangeline, who died of typhoid fever when she was only five years old.

Dr. Northrup and his wife had passed away by the time we moved to Markle, but Mary and I have one of Eva Northrup's original oil paintings on our wall. Lillian McGuffey gave it to me years ago when I was visiting her on a house call. In this painting, two sailboats struggle to stay afloat on a frothy, storm-vexed sea. It's a dark painting, and I wonder what year Mrs. Northrup painted it, whether it portrays the inner turmoil she and her husband must have felt after the death of their only child.

Few Markle residents still recognize the name of Dr. Ernest C. Fishbaugh, though he is probably the town's most famous native son. That's because when he was a young man Dr. Fishbaugh decided to move away from Markle and practice medicine in Beverly Hills.

Ernest was born in Markle to Rufus and Rosella Fishbaugh in 1884 and received his first twelve years of schooling at Markle Public School. According to the *Huntington Herald*, Ernest graduated from high school in 1904 and attended commencement in the "densely packed" Markle Opera House. This opera house was above a store, but any crowded space is noteworthy when you consider that there were only four graduates and two of them were siblings—Ernest and his brother Clarence. "Aim High," was the class motto and Ernest, the valedictorian, apparently took it to heart. In 1913 he graduated from John Hopkins Medical School and was recommended as a House Officer (an intern at John Hopkins) based on his outstanding academic performance.

In 1914 Dr. Fishbaugh and his first wife moved to California where the doctor became a preeminent Hollywood doctor and surgeon. He developed a hugely successful practice in Beverly Hills and served as an Assistant Professor in the Medical Department of the University of Southern California. Nowadays, Dr. Fishbaugh is mostly remembered as being Jean Harlow's personal physician and the doctor treating her when she died at age twenty-six of edema caused by kidney failure. Most likely the actress' kidneys were irreparably damaged as a result of contracting scarlet fever when she was a teenager. Four days before her death Dr. Fishbaugh told reporters that Miss Harlow had a cold, but that might have been at the actress' bidding. Even if he had suspected the problem was with her kidneys, he couldn't have saved her life—not in 1937, without antibiotics, dialysis, or a kidney transplant option.

Dr. Fishbaugh was also in the headlines a decade earlier when two of his Beverly Hills patients died in one of the most controversial murder mysteries of the early twentieth century. Police investigators concluded that Ned Doheny, the son of Edward L. Doheny, a powerful oil tycoon, was shot by Hugh Plunkett, his friend and secretary. Plunkett apparently asked the young Doheny for a raise, and when he refused, Plunkett shot him and then in remorse killed himself.

I'm drawn to any kind of mystery so this one easily intrigues me. Both young men were going to be called up for Congressional questioning in the infamous Teapot Dome Scandal, a bribery incident in which national oil reserves were leased to Edward Doheny and Harry Sinclair without competitive bidding. Investigators never explored the possibility that fear of Plunkett's upcoming testimony might have been a motive for his murder. Ned Doheny and Dr. Fishbaugh had recently tried without success to convince Plunkett he was on the verge of a nervous breakdown and should enter a sanitarium. The other witness to the bribery scandal was conveniently confined to an asylum at the time of the trial.

Key details of Dr. Fishbaugh's first version of events, such as his denial that he ever moved Doheny's body before the police arrived, contradict his later accounts. Detective novelist Raymond Chandler believed that Ned Doheny killed Plunkett and then himself. His first novel, *High Window,* includes a digression that refers to the case and a cover up that included the district attorney and family doctor.

Ned Doheny's parents paid for their only son, as well as the man who supposedly murdered him, to be buried in Glendale's exclusive Forest Lawn Park Memorial. Eventually, Dr. Fishbaugh was buried there, too, eighteen hundred miles from the Wabash.

I wonder how Markle history might have been different if Dr. Fishbaugh had practiced medicine in his own hometown. What if, like George Bailey in *It's a Wonderful Life,* he had decided his small town needed him too much to leave it? What if he had worked from an office on Morse Street and used his considerable surgical skills in Huntington and Bluffton? What changes would he have initiated? How would he have made a difference in his hometown community? Why would he be remembered?

ON THE SIDELINES

One of the ways Lee and I socialized with the community was through our voluntary work as team physicians for Norwell High School. Right away, we became staunch fans, attending football and basketball games at home and away.

Our families arrived in Markle just as Northern Wells County was consolidating four township high schools: East Rock Creek, East Union, Jefferson, and Lancaster. Students at the new Norwell High School now had more classes to choose from, as well as sports. Previously, the township schools never had enough athletes or funding for a football program, but now, as a larger school, Norwell began developing a team. This wasn't easy since the boys hadn't grown up playing football. We had some hefty players who looked impressive as they charged out to the field. However, when the game started, their opponents plowed over them. Our inexperienced players often overreacted to small injuries, even minor bumps and bruises. So those first several years, Lee and I were especially busy along the sidelines.

With such lop-sided game scores, Knight fans tended to be fair-weather. At one away game during the second year, it began raining midway through the third quarter, and when I glanced around, I realized the only other fans on our side of the field were two fathers and my friend, Jerry Mossburg, from Huntington County. As seventh and eighth graders started playing football, Norwell gradually started winning some games.

By the time Lee and Dawn's youngest son, Matthew, joined Norwell's football roster in 1978, the team was considerably better. Matt went on to Purdue University where he set a punting record. Like his father, he was a talented baseball pitcher, pitching a season with the St. Louis Cardinals and a game with the Detroit Tigers. He also punted a game for the Detroit Lions, earning him the nickname "The Detroit Liger" and the distinction of the only person to have played for the Lions and the Tigers. Since then, two Norwell graduates have played on NFL teams— Jeff Miller for the Chicago Bears and Chandler Harnish for the Indianapolis Colts.

At Norwell, as at most Indiana high schools, Hoosier Hysteria is endemic and fans flock to basketball games whether or not the team is having a winning season. I enjoyed watching the games every year, but Norwell's 1972-73 boys basketball season, when Shari was a freshman, still stands out as special. Half-way through the season, as we were winning over some larger schools, pep blocks across the gym floor started denouncing our boys as "Farmers." Though they meant this as an insult, our fans turned it into a compliment. We started wearing flannel shirts and overalls and sporting bandanas. Local dry good and hardware stores couldn't keep up with this demand for agricultural apparel— especially the desire for bandanas. Fans tied red and blue handkerchiefs around their necks or wore them as headscarves. They sported them from overall pockets. They waved them whenever our team made a basket or needed a quick boost of support.

The cheers grew deafening as our Farmers won sectional and then regional. As in the film *Hoosiers*, intense excitement and pride pulled people together. This was before class basketball when you could still have an upset as amazing as the 1954 Milan Miracle, when a school with an enrollment of only 161 won the state championship. Norwell was four times the size of Milan, but it was still exciting to see our team go as far as a game in the state semi-finals before bowing to Concord High School in Elkhart, a much larger school.

Hoosier Hysteria was all about boys' basketball until 1976 when Title IX required schools to offer equal educational opportunities regardless of gender. A one-class Indiana State Girls Basketball Tournament was instituted that year, and from the start Norwell girls had the talent and coaching to be a contender. By the team's second year, it had developed a strong following and excitement grew intense as tourney time approached. Families—including ours—placed signs and banners along State Route 224 to show support and encourage a winning attitude. The girls kept winning every Saturday as they advanced toward Indianapolis, and eventually they took runner-up in the Final Four.

That season our amazing point guard Terri Rosinski was awarded the title of Miss Indiana Basketball. It's unusual for a school to have a second winner, but it happened again in 2012 when Jessica Rupright received the distinction.

Although Lee and I were never team physicians for Huntington North High School, we still rooted for their athletes and felt community pride in 1996 when a Viking, Lisa Winter, received the Miss Basketball title. After all, more than half of our town was in Huntington County and many of our friends and patients lived there.

Of course, years ago, there was neither Knight nor Viking. Teams from Markle's brick schoolhouse were called the Eagles. Before that, they had a moniker that might have caused rival schools to underestimate their potential. At least that's the only benefit I can see in touting themselves the Markle Midgets.

A WALK THROUGH THE INN

Under Mary's creative guidance, the Markle Church of the Brethren transformed each year into the Inn of Bethlehem. On the first Sunday evening after Thanksgiving, electricity was turned off. Kerosene lamps and candles were lit. Visitors from as far away as Fort Wayne entered the basement where they were assigned to a tribe of Israel and given a census card. They sat at tables snacking on coffee, hot chocolate, cookies, and dried fruit, as they waited for a guide to appear.

Every year for eleven years I put on a robe, sandals, a curly wig, and a beard to become one of these guides. From the onset I took to this role. It was my favorite of any I played in the church dramas Mary directed. I liked playing Zacchaeus, but it was painful to have to walk on my knees. When I played him and other characters, including a disciple in *The Last Supper* and a deceased church member tethered to my grave (a la *Our Town*), I had to stick to my lines, but as a guide through the inn I could insert ad libs into the script. I enjoyed interacting with my groups, each one named for a tribe of Israel.

Everywhere we went—to the innkeeper's office, the cookery, a rabbi's classroom, the apothecary, and mercantile shop—we listened to other characters and always caught some passing reference to a Galilean couple who had arrived earlier that night. As we strolled through the dimly-lit hallways, I had to warn members of my group to keep a tight grip on their census cards; without those cards the Roman soldiers performing random checks would throw them into the jailhouse. Now and then a beggar would trail us, crying out, "Alms for the poor! Alms for the poor!" Every year he wore the same tattered fur coat someone had found in their barn—or maybe it just smelled that way. Our event was free so what the beggar collected in his tin cup went toward meeting the evening's expenses and helping any community members in need.

We followed a group of shepherds outdoors to find a bright star perched in a tree branch above a tent donated and set up each year by Everett Wilson's Burial Vaults. Inside, amid bales of stacked straw, stood some local sheep, a donkey, and, one year, a llama. These animals were always mute—maybe they were stage struck—in any case, to make the scene more realistic, Mary had dubbed her own intermittent bleats and brays into a taped reading of the Christmas story that Joseph could click to play and then rewind behind the manger. Flickering candles lodged in pots of sand illumined him, his wife, and their newborn son.

When you're part of a small town like Markle, you have the opportunity to do things you wouldn't otherwise do if you knew there were more qualified people who could take your place. We needed the factory worker at K & K Tool to play the rabbi, the banker to shine a spotlight from the balcony on the soldiers, two public school teachers to take the census, a dairy farmer to portray the beggar, a homemaker to be a guide, any young, naive couple (who hadn't foreseen how cold it would be standing outside on a night in late November) to play Mary and Joseph.

For one evening a year, we used our imaginations to usher the long ago past into the present moment. Then our church took on double duty as a daycare center, and after that there was no room for the inn.

A LARGER WORLD

Vera's Gateway Inn was one of my favorite Markle restaurants. Located on Road 3, just north of the railroad tracks, it served delicious broasted chicken and homemade mashed potatoes with noodles. The décor, though, was ordinary—just a counter with chrome stools and lots of booths until it was bought by a local man who was also an avid hunter. The food still remained about the same, but he added some ambiance by building on a smoke-free family dining area he decorated with stuffed wildlife. Customers could enjoy a fried fish dinner next to a mounted sailfish or an ermine poised on a branch. They could dine under a gray hornet hive or the gaze of an antelope or coyote. Sometimes there were pheasants or a red fox. I don't remember all of the animals; they kept changing.

Though Gateway Inn is no longer open, the owner's penchant for wild décor will not soon be forgotten. If you speak with older residents of the community or peruse past issues of the *Markle Times*, you rapidly realize that the people honored in town history are those with interesting hobbies or idiosyncrasies.

For instance, I never knew Hod Sparks, but I know that he was an exceptional fisherman who carried his bait—live crawfish—directly on his bald head and under his hat.

I did know Kenneth McBride. He drove a milk route but is better remembered for playing three instruments well and all at one time. Kenneth played saxophone with his left hand, strummed a banjo with his right, and worked a drum with his foot. He formed a two-man band with his brother, Ralph, who blew into a kazoo while fingering a piano with his right hand and plucking a banjo with his left.

When the Markle Medical Center was downtown, I could look across the street to see Siamese cats staring at me through the window of the dry clean delivery service. Sometimes a diapered monkey gazed through the plate glass, too. These animals were real, and they belonged to a businesswoman fondly called *The Monkey Woman*. To my best knowledge, she had only one monkey, but I don't know how many Siamese cats she owned. I was just inside her home once, and during that visit I noticed more cats peering down at me from the bookshelves.

As doctors and nurses, we had our idiosyncrasies, too. I liked to freshen the air with a squirt of the drug Camerol. Dr. Joe Greene would fill an ear syringe with water, prime it, and shoot the staff between the eyes. Katherine, our head nurse, doodled a lot. She didn't draw on charts—but on any loose scrap of paper. Dr. Deborah Miller would bring injured animals into the office—any chipmunk, bird, rabbit, or other wild creature she found hurt along the road.

The idiosyncrasies of certain patients also made days in the office more interesting. The nurses seemed to notice these more than I did. One woman would hum all of the time— maybe it helped her control her nerves or she was just happy to see us. One elderly man always flirted with the nurses, asking them over and over again if they were married. Another older farmer wore so many layers of clothing that the nurses had a hard time taking his blood pressure. When this man paid for a visit, instead of pulling money from a wallet, he pulled it from between the strata of his clothes.

Appreciation for the uniqueness of individuals has a long tradition in Markle and is evident in the assignation of affectionate nicknames like *The Monkey Woman*. From an article Eldon Wolf wrote in the *Markle Times*, I learned that *Poodle* (Carl Brandt) took his pet poodle everywhere he went. *P-Nuckle* (Leorice Brian) liked to play pinochle so much that it was one of his favorite topics of conversation. In his youth *Mounty* (Harold Will) enjoyed trying to imitate the physical feats of the Canadian Royal Mounted Police he watched in movies and read about in books. Even in the winter, *Frosty* (Don Wolf) drove his 1941 Buick with the windows down so he could relish the roar of his altered exhaust system. Apparently *Sly* (Jay Fox) gained his nickname just because it went so well with *Fox*.

Some of the town's more distinctive residents, like Oren *Pappy* Johnson, might have lived lonely, difficult lives in other settings, but Markle residents accepted their differences and looked out for them. When I knew him late in his life, Oren had Parkinson's, but from his birth in 1910, he contended with other physical disabilities, possibly as the result of cerebral palsy. Townspeople remembered he had always walked with a slight stagger and that his hands shook. Each weekday at 11 o'clock he'd walk straight down the middle of the street to the center of town, looking for someone to offer him work. Someone almost always did. Storekeepers and farmers would pay him to do odd jobs, and whenever anyone died, the undertaker hired him to excavate the grave with his hand shovel and pick. Marilyn Mason, who grew up next door to Oren, remembered her mother inviting him to their supper table and taking him meals.

Oren didn't let Parkinson's alter his positive outlook on life. Lee told me that when he saw Oren outside, he would pick him up for some good company as he drove to a house call.

In a town as small as Markle, even those who won't or can't march in step have a place in the parade. Or another way to look at it—everyone has a part in the drama.

One story from the annals of town history sounds like it could have been a plot for an episode of the old *Andy Griffith Show*. This anecdote takes place in 1936 when the town decided to stage a play in order to raise funds for the Markle Fish and Game Club. Phyllis Haflich, as the pianist, was the only woman in the cast of Wendell Hite's *Ladies for a Night*. The other forty-five cast members were men who played the parts of females. Though gender-specific, this large cast represented a cross-section of occupations: the town veterinarian, police officer, mechanic, barber, and more.

Phyllis recalled one cast member worrying excessively about the pronunciation of *succor* in the line, "Is there no succor for a damsel in distress?"

On performance night he panicked, blurting out a line befitting Barney Fife's strained falsetto voice: "Won't some sucker help a damsel in distress?"

British author G.K. Chesterton once wrote: "The man who lives in a small community lives in a much larger world. He knows much more of the fierce variety and uncompromising divergences of men." He explains that in a large community we can choose our companions, but in a small community those companions are chosen for us.

"There is nothing really narrow about the clan," he notes; "the thing which is really narrow is the clique."

A HARD DOOR TO OPEN

I greatly valued the sense of belonging I felt as part of a close-knit community, but there were times when such closeness made my work as a physician more difficult. Giving friends and neighbors a sad prognosis or speaking to them after a loss was more stressful than if those patients had been only acquaintances. Medical school hadn't really prepared me for the emotional challenges of treating people who were also my friends. My residency in Fort Wayne hadn't either. When I worked in the emergency rooms at Lutheran Hospital, I sometimes had the hard task of speaking to family members after an unexpected death, but that was made easier by the fact that I didn't know the deceased or their families.

One of my most difficult challenges occurred in July of 1965 when I had been in Markle for seventeen months. I still remember opening the door to Marjorie Caley's hospital room. That door was hard to push open—not because it was heavy, but due to the depth of grief on the other side. As I entered it was if I were walking into water over my head, there was such deep sorrow and dim light. Because bright light worsened my patient's headache, the curtains were drawn and only a small lamp illuminated the room.

Near the bedside, I pulled up a chair.

Marjorie turned her head to look at me. "Did they suffer?"

My answer, though reassuring, still remained harsh: "No, they all died at the moment of impact."

In the muted light what kept flashing before Marjorie's eyes was the previous Tuesday evening, when a car ran a four-way stop at high speed, broadsiding her family's sedan. She landed in a cornfield, with a fractured pelvis and some minor injuries, but the rest of the Caley family, her husband and four children, died in the crash.

As Marjorie's general practitioner, I could care for her fracture, but how could I help heal her grief? How could I speak to her as a doctor and a friend?

Marjorie and her husband, Bill, served on the search committee that asked Lee and me to come to Markle. Even before we moved they made us feel welcome by inviting our families to their home for an afternoon of swimming and a poolside meal. When Lee and I had questions about the community, the Caleys were some of the first people we turned to for information and counsel. This couple knew the community well since they were active in church and local service clubs. In fact, Bill's family had farmed in Wells County for more than a hundred years. His great-great-grandfather, Samuel Caley, moved to the area from Ohio in the early 1840s, when a Miami village stood just across the river from land that would later be Markle.

Sometimes, beyond all probability, one tragedy links to another with a hard twist. Six years earlier, Bill's father, mother, aunt, and uncle were all killed at the same intersection, just three miles east of Markle, where Indiana 116 and 303 cross. In that accident, two teenagers playing chicken with their car lights off ran the stop sign and hit Clifford and Cressie Caley's car. The Caleys and Hafliches were traveling home from the Bluffton Street Fair.

Bill and Marjorie's family were en route to the Wells County 4-H Fair. The children—Kevin, Kriss, Kent, and Kirby—were all planning to show their livestock that night. I am sure that as they drove toward the fair an atmosphere of excitement pervaded the car. This family was passionate about 4-H, and as a former 4-H member myself, we shared an enthusiasm for that organization. Like the Caley kids, I raised a calf each year to show at my county fair.

In another ironic twist of fate, I injured Kirby's 4-H calf the year before, during my first summer in Markle. I was driving to the office from early morning hospital rounds when the young steer broke out of the barnyard and darted across my path. Kevin, thirteen years old at the time, understood when the wounded animal had to be shot. He remained my friend and appreciated how badly I felt about the accident. It pained me to think of how his dreams had been dashed.

Now everything seemed dashed. I truthfully told Marjorie that her family didn't suffer, that death was instantaneous. I also spoke from my heart to assure her that Bill and her children would be waiting to meet her at the end of her life. This last reassurance was not what a doctor is expected to say, but I was not just Marjorie's doctor, I was also her friend. Then I took time to sit with her because sometimes just being with a friend is more meaningful than any words.

The next day I would see that the most effective medicine is practiced within a caring community. Marjorie's true healing began as she traveled west on Morse Street where every store was closed for the funeral. The medical office was closed, too. Lee and I accompanied Marjorie as she was wheeled into the crowded church on a cot. Friends and neighbors pressed her shoulder and held her hand. We let her know we were with her. It's what a community does.

LORI ANN

Of course, no matter how caring, no community is immune from the possibility of violence. One bitter cold March we discovered that one of our youth, a thirteen-year-old girl, had been murdered.

I'm aware of only one other homicide in the Markle vicinity. It's not well-documented, but purportedly happened many years ago, possibly in the 1800s. That body wasn't discovered in Markle, but two miles west of Rock Creek Center, near the William Bowman farm, by a spring which purportedly never froze. The victim was a well-to-do peddler who had been selling his wares in the area. No one was ever charged for the murder and the legend developed that the ground near the spring was haunted. At night odd lights and floating specters would suddenly appear and then vanish.

Lori Ann Brickley's murder has never been solved either. She disappeared on the evening of Monday, March 18, 1974. She walked downtown from her home to run a few errands for her family but never returned. After buying a few items at the corner drugstore, at about 8:40, Lori was last seen entering the alley north of Morse Street, apparently taking a short cut to the post office before returning home. It was dark by then, especially in the alley, but people in town didn't worry much about safety. Doors were often left unlocked at night and children freely walked or rode their bikes about town. Lori lived up the hill from downtown, along State Route 224 or Logan Street, the same street our family lived on our first year in town. When news surfaced the next day that Lori was missing, the whole town was worried.

Lori attended Salamonie Junior High in Huntington County and liked to play sports, especially basketball. Townspeople described her to reporters as "warm and friendly" and "tomboyish." One resident said she was athletic and could "run like a deer." Lori liked to play basketball and was a member of the Girls Athletic Association at school. Town Marshal Rex Sprowl and Lori's parents never believed that Lori had run away because there hadn't been any indication of problems at home or at school.

Over the next few days Markle hosted Huntington County Police, the Indiana State Police, and even FBI agents. Officers traced and retraced Lori's path from the drugstore to the post office and then uphill toward her home, but they found no evidence of any struggle. At least thirty townspeople helped the police look for clues. Schoolchildren combed the shoreline along Huntington Lake and searched through town buildings. Finally, on Thursday, between 4 and 4:30 p.m., Ivan Ormsby, a seventy-four-year-old neighbor helping with the search, saw Lori's body through a missing plank in an outhouse door. This shed was directly behind an old abandoned house on Logan Street, a house which was padlocked and only three doors down from Lori's home.

An autopsy revealed that Lori had died of a stab wound to the upper left chest that penetrated an artery. She had, in fact, been stabbed multiple times and mutilated. Although there were blood stains on the outhouse floorboards, investigators theorized that the murder took place elsewhere and the body hidden afterward in the shed. The next morning, on Friday, officers found Lori's package from the drugstore. It was against the side of the abandoned house, hidden under a layer of early spring snow.

Lori's brutal death was a tragedy that stunned our community. It brought us together in our grief for her, as well as for her parents and five siblings. With the possibility that the murderer was still nearby, there was also an atmosphere of apprehension that lasted for months. Doors seldom locked were now secured, and children playing outdoors were supervised. Sporadically during those first months of investigation, State Police detectives stopped by the medical office to ask me for history on several residents in town. They told me they thought the murderer was a local person and that they would soon solve the case.

But the months passed and then years. Lori's murder is a cold case, still waiting to be solved.

THE MARKLE TIMES

Mary devoted much of her time to supporting community activities. Besides directing dramas at our church and chairing or co-chairing the Markle Wildcat Festival, she started a Red Hat Society and was a member of the women's service group, Psi Iota Xi (affectionately nicknamed the "Psi Otes" or "Coyotes"). With her bookkeeping skills, Mary also served for many years as Treasurer of the Markle Business and Community Association and later, the Markle Chamber of Commerce. But maybe her greatest achievement was helping to create ninety-three issues of the *Markle Times*.

This monthly newspaper was launched in 1997 following a series of discussions between Ball State students and the Markle Business and Community Association. Hired to study our town and then give ideas for revitalizing it, the group came up with these suggestions:

1. Employ a town manager to co-ordinate upcoming projects.
2. Improve the sewer system so that a twenty-year ban on new growth can be lifted.
3. Take advantage of the Wabash River by enhancing the appearance of the bridge and developing the riverside land through trails and other development.
4. Make the downtown more attractive by adding a sidewalk lined with brick pavers and new lighting.
5. Add a new sign, playground equipment, and a pavilion shelter to the Markle Fish & Game Park.
6. Reestablish a local grade school that can also serve as a community center.

7. Add new housing to establish a larger tax base.

8. Start a town newspaper.

The Markle Business and Community Association got busy and everything on this list was accomplished—except for the development of the riverside land and the reestablishment of a local grade school. I liked that idea of trails and some eateries along the waterway—I've seen some towns that have successfully done that—but no one stepped forward to take leadership in what would mean considerable time spent in making plans and procuring grants.

Seventy-five percent of Markle residents were in favor of a local grade school and one townsperson even offered to donate the land, but, unfortunately, the proposal failed to gain approval from the Northern Wells School Board. Still, the town accomplished much within the space of just a few years. A momentum for improvement was sparked that led some downtown businesses to remodel and some new ones to move in. An unattractive downtown parking area that had been the site of an A&W drive-in when we first moved to Markle, soon became Veterans' Park, with a white gazebo, two millstones, and a pedestal clock.

The new monthly newspaper, *Markle Times,* garnered support for revitalization efforts by conveying the purpose of the projects and what the public could do to help. The Markle Business and Community Association financially supported the first issue which appeared on October 1997. After that, business ads covered the cost of free mailings to all the townspeople and residents of the surrounding rural area. Issues were usually twenty pages in length, but no one on the staff, including the editor, was ever paid, so that held down expenses. During the first year, Barbara Oldham served as editor, aided by a staff that included Mary. Along with several others, Mary wrote or secured news stories and collected money for ads. After the first year, Barbara had to retire from her position for health reasons, so Mary and Lydia Kahlenbeck took over as co-editors. Two years later, when Lydia started a full-time job, Mary assumed full editorship.

The paper's stated purpose was to bring together the past, the present, and the future—and it met that goal in every issue. Details about the upcoming Grouch Contest might be followed by a description and photo of the new downtown park; a historical account of Markle's first settlers might be next to information about the opening of a floral shop or improvements to the sewer system.

I helped with this paper, too. Each month I contributed an advice column, "To Your Health." In my articles I shared recent medical news or made suggestions for healthier living. Educating the community on health issues was not a new endeavor for me. The teacher in me always enjoyed reaching out to people beyond the context of an office visit. Over the years I gave talks related to health at schools and churches, and for about eight years prior to writing my column I had a radio spot called "House Calls" on the Fort Wayne Christian Radio Station, WBLC. The news director prerecorded the sessions at my home during the lunch hour, yet they were always rather stressful for me since I knew that once the tape was on its way from my home to the radio station I couldn't call it back. Writing for the newspaper was less stressful and just as rewarding.

My favorite articles to read in the *Markle Times* were the historical pieces, many of them contributed by Reada Espich, a member of the Markle Historical Society, and Eldon Wolf, a former Markle resident who lived in Wisconsin. I also especially enjoyed the personal profiles of individuals or couples, written to mark a significant anniversary or to stand as a memorial after they died.

I found it fascinating how one article about a person or event in Markle's history would set off a chain-reaction of stories. For example, in Issue 54 Eldon related a boyhood encounter with Civil War veteran William (Billy) Earhart that inspired others to share what they knew about this man. Eldon described how one afternoon in 1935 he was crouched on the brick sidewalk in front of his house, digging out grass with his pocketknife, when a "stately old neighbor" walked up to him. He asked Eldon if he would like a story to tell his teacher and schoolmates the next day. When he said he would, the old man told him he had been a messenger in the Union Army and one rainy night had a particularly important sealed message to deliver. The message was for President Lincoln. When the guard at the President's tent said he'd take the letter, William told him his orders were to deliver the message in person and to wait for a reply. "You may not see the President now for he is in prayer," said the guard, "but you may step into the foyer and wait for him to finish."

"I stepped into the foyer and, to be sure, the President was in prayer at great length," said William. "As I stood there seeing him on his knees, it left a permanent image on my mind. The message was read, answered, and sealed in an envelope, and I rode off into the darkness."

Five issues later, Eldon wrote that Bob Randol read his article and told him that Billy lived directly across the street from him. He was a house painter who operated from a push cart, and many of his eight sons were painters, too. In that same article, Eldon also provided information he gleaned from Billy's great-grandson. This man from Fort Wayne was passing through Markle when he stopped at the Davis Restaurant and picked up an issue of *Markle Times.* As he scanned the ads for antiques, he was surprised to find an article about his great-grandfather.

He told Eldon that a local farmer, Jacob Lesh, paid Billy five hundred dollars to take his place in the Union Army. While serving with the C-40 Company of Indiana, Billy was shot twice, but neither wound was serious. One grazed his head and another cut through the straps on his backpack. Billy died in 1937, at age ninety-two.

The next month's issue had a photograph of Billy and carried more information—this time written by the great-grandson himself. Paul Hanauer had firsthand memories of his great-grandfather and remembered seeing his complete uniform and gun. "He got a pension of $100 a month," Paul wrote, "and after he died, the boys found hundred dollar bills rolled up in the blinds all over the house."

These stories about Billy inspired more stories about Markle veterans. For instance, Hubert Girvin wrote that when his father was wounded in World War I, official notification was sent that he had died. Forest Girvin's mother had a wonderful shock one day when the son she was mourning walked into the house.

One of the best things about our local paper was how it connected people who had moved away from town with people who still lived there. Sometimes it even connected people to Markle who had never resided there themselves.

One reader, a doctor in a distant state, never lived in Markle, but his relatives did. When he read my daughter Shari's article about the condition of the cemetery, he wrote that it touched him deeply. "I think often of that small plot of sacred land and its current state," he wrote. "Having buried my father there this winter, I am all too conscious of the encroachment of commercialism and lack of a coordinated vision." This man, who wished to remain anonymous, donated a considerable amount of money to the Cemetery Association so that it could add a pine tree border, shade trees, benches, and a re-designed entrance.

It's interesting to note that in the early 1900s Markle supported two concurrent newspapers: *Markle Journal*, founded in 1892, and *The Gazette*, created in 1913. Those commercial papers disappeared long before we moved to town. For decades there was no town paper until the advent of the *Markle Times*. When Mary retired after nine years of working on the paper, a local graphic and design marketing company tried to keep it alive as a commercial venture, but that attempt was short-lived.

Looking back, Mary says what she misses most about working on the *Markle Times* is the morning each month when she'd meet with others to fold and tape the papers for mailing. Bette Brane and Alfreda and Jean Mossburg were regulars, but other retired women helped, too, and sometimes a few older men. These meetings were a time of laughter, of sharing town news and maybe some gossip. As volunteers attached address labels they often gave Mary suggestions for future stories. To celebrate the send-off of another issue, the group lunched at Davis Restaurant or Dairy Queen or The Pickle.

When I consider what the *Markle Times* accomplished—garnering enthusiasm for downtown renovation, preserving town history, honoring the dead and the living, connecting community members near and far, I realize the wisdom of those Ball State students when they listed a town newspaper as a step toward a revitalized community.

FIVE: THE BEST MEDICINE

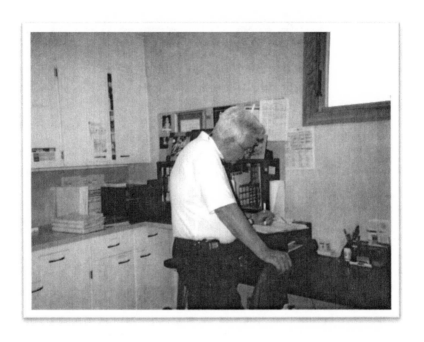

THE ART OF THE OFFICE VISIT

"When I go to the doctor, he doesn't listen. He's always in a hurry." That was a complaint I often heard from patients. Or they would say, "My doctor doesn't seem to care much about my problems; he only wants to take care of what he thinks is important." Sometimes I heard, "I wish I could tell my doctor how I really feel."

Such comments would be rare if doctors recognized some key components of a good office visit. Learning a patient's history is a primary one. Since gathering a history is so important, I found it necessary that the first appointment with a patient be longer, so as to gather adequate information. Our office appointments were scheduled in fifteen minute increments, and for each new patient, I usually reserved two to four of these time blocks.

This history not only includes the patient's medical history; it entails background concerning his or her family, social network, and work environment. One life story is a part of other life stories, and in a rural community like Markle those stories form a granary of narratives that nourish understanding. I agree with Wendell Berry in *The Art of the Commonplace* when he says that "the community — in the fullest sense: a place and all its creatures — is the smallest unit of health and that to speak of the health of an isolated individual is a contradiction in terms."

It didn't take Lee and me long to observe that in the Markle community there were some diseases that ran in families and, since many of the families had a long history of living in the Wells and Huntington area, the affected families were quite extensive. Certain families had a high incidence of breast cancer, and we could target early detection in those extended families to improve the survival rate. This was a new approach back in the 1960s. The same was true with heart disease, diabetes, and hyperlipidemia as we discovered families with members predisposed to developing those diseases at a young age. We worked at decreasing their risk factors and getting them to a specialist for early intervention.

But not all diseases linked to heredity could be predicted by knowing the past. A few diseases seemed to appear suddenly in a family, and then Lee and I knew to check other members and to keep an eye on succeeding generations. The most dramatic incident involved a disease that to the best of our knowledge had not appeared in that family, at least not within their memory. Acoustic neuroma is a rather rare disease and generally not even considered hereditary. An acoustic neuroma is a tumor that develops at the base of the eighth cranial nerve, the nerve that extends from the brain to each ear and helps with hearing and balance. Acoustic neuroma's early symptoms may be decreased hearing in the affected ear, vertigo, and headaches.

The first patient we diagnosed, with the help of a neurologist, was a teenage girl. Soon the girl's mother developed similar symptoms. Eventually, one of the sons was also discovered to have acoustic neuroma and so was his cousin. The neurosurgeon in Fort Wayne who removed the tumors thought this might be the largest family ever discovered with acoustic neuroma.

The son had a tumor removed from one acoustic nerve and seven years later from the other nerve. That left him with total deafness. He also had some facial paralysis because the facial nerve lies so close to the acoustic nerve. My patient went to rehabilitation to learn new ways to balance and walk. Eventually, he learned to lip read and because of lower facial muscle paralysis, how to speak again, too. The Markle community and his church assisted him in many ways but, most importantly, by helping him find local jobs he could do without the sense of hearing. His mother and sister both died from their disease, but, fortunately, he was cured.

My experience with this family made me much more aware of acoustic neuroma and later helped me diagnose two other patients with this rare disease, none of whom were related to the family. One underwent surgery at the Mayo Clinic, and the other is just being observed since the individual is older and the tumor slow-growing.

Families not only share genes—they share some of the same environmental risk factors. A new patient once came to me who complained of severe fatigue. She said she was becoming increasingly tired and had been to several doctors for this problem. They had determined she was anemic and given her iron tablets and shots. Still, she wasn't getting better. I noticed her pallor and inquired if anyone else at home was pale. When she mentioned that her teenage daughter also complained of being tired, I asked the patient to bring all three of her children to the office to be tested for anemia.

As it turned out, they were all anemic. This suggested that the anemia was caused by an environmental factor and that I could ascertain the source of my patient's problem through questions—instead of running more tests. When I asked about the family's diet and other family history, I didn't hear anything out of the ordinary. But when I asked about poisons, I discovered that for two years she had been placing mothballs in drawers—dresser drawers, desk drawers, kitchen drawers, even the silverware drawer—because she liked how they smelled. Naphthalene, an aromatic, white crystalline solid, is the main ingredient in mothballs, and exposure to large amounts can damage or destroy red blood cells, causing hemolytic anemia. My patient removed the mothballs from her home, and within several months the whole family was back to normal—substantially energized.

Establishing rapport with a patient is also important in any office visit. I tried to look at the patient with interest and to appear relaxed even when other pressing matters were competing for space in my mind or when a recent emergency had moved us behind in our schedule. Stories and comments I heard from patients confirmed the need to not appear in a hurry.

In 1970 when I accepted a year's term as an interim doctor at a Mennonite hospital in Somalia, I urged a married couple who lived in Huntertown, thirty miles north of Markle, that they begin seeing a doctor closer to home during my absence. They made an appointment with a physician in Fort Wayne, but, upon returning from Africa, I found the couple back in my office. I asked how they had gotten along with their new doctor while I was away.

"He was always in a hurry," they said. "When he entered the room, he was ready to leave. He never took his hand off the doorknob. Even when he listened to our heart, he kept one hand on the doorknob." I'm sure that at some point the doctor removed his hand from the knob, but this habit was his way of controlling the appointment.

In order to develop a strong relationship with patients, it helps if doctors explain what they're doing during an examination. In later years, when our practice had grown, we had one doctor who had trouble establishing rapport with his patients. For example, people would complain that they saw him for a cough but that he never listened to their chest. This doctor would have charted what he heard and so certainly did examine the patient—but he didn't make it a notable exam. Because patients don't always understand what is going on in an exam and can easily forget that I checked them, I learned to tell patients what I was doing at each step and what I discovered: "Now I'm listening to your heart. The rhythm is normal and I hear no murmurs. . . .Now I'm listening to your lungs so take a slow, deep breath." The exam doesn't take any longer, but it focuses the patient's attention so he sees, hears, and remembers what you are doing.

During an effective office call, a doctor respects a patient's chief complaint. Our nurses would jot down a sentence at the beginning of each visit describing the principal complaint in the patient's own words. We wanted to take care of that complaint no matter how insignificant it appeared. Patients might have other problems more medically pressing, but this complaint was important to them and needed to be addressed.

Writing down the chief complaint could be helpful for subsequent visits. When patients came in for their next appointment, I would ask, "How do you feel?" They might say, "I'm no better." But when I would then read back their main physical complaint from the previous appointment, they'd often respond, "Oh, that has gone away. I don't have that anymore."

Although a doctor should address the patient's principal complaint, he or she should also strive to see the whole picture when analyzing symptoms. Patients often have a number of symptoms that they want the doctor to approach one at a time. But the ailment that best helps diagnose the problem may be the one they mention just before the end of the appointment. So for patients with multiple symptoms, I would ask that they list all of these on a piece of paper before coming to the office. When they handed me the list, I could then pose better-informed questions. Several symptoms were usually related, and then I could group them as one problem that we could address during the appointment. This process saved a lot of time and allowed me to provide much better medical care.

In a society in which time is money and people multi-task while checking a wristwatch or the clock on their iPhone, I can see how internet office calls can be tempting — especially when skyping allows a doctor to actually look at the patient. I often made a diagnosis from a visual examination, sometimes in the first three minutes of an office call. I'd see the typical lesions of shingles — Herpes Zoster, for example — and make a swift diagnosis. However, during the rest of the appointment, after I'd explained the disease and discussed the treatment, I would also examine the patient for any underlying problems.

For instance, one sixty-five-year-old woman came to the office with a small area of skin lesions typical of shingles. After explaining the cause and treatment of this disease, I asked her to stand while I did a quick physical examination. When I felt her abdomen, I was surprised to detect a large mass. She had a huge spleen that filled her left side. Within several days we knew that, in addition to shingles, this woman had chronic lymphocytic leukemia. If I had only treated her over the phone or internet without examining more than her rash, treatment would have been delayed. As it was, a few extra minutes of my time gave my patient extra years.

DETECTIVE SKILLS

I enjoy reading about medical mysteries from the past. One such mystery took place in and around New York City in the early 1900s. For six years typhoid fever struck a series of wealthy households and no pattern was discovered until a doctor, George Soper, figured out that the households had all hired the same cook—a hot-tempered Irish-American named Mary Mallon. *Typhoid Mary*, as she was eventually called, admitted that she never washed her hands before cooking, but she denied any possible culpability since she was perfectly healthy. When Dr. Soper asked for a stool sample, she brandished a meat cleaver, but eventually a sample was obtained and it provided ample proof that Mary was indeed infected by typhoid bacteria.

Though not as dramatic, I've had some interesting medical mysteries to solve, too. One involved a factory worker who lived near Markle with his wife and two children. This man enjoyed raising some livestock and tending a large vegetable garden. One August day his wife brought him to the office after he had suffered three days of explosive and persistent diarrhea. He also had a low-grade fever and looked much more ill than you'd expect from someone sick for only three days. He had lost ten pounds and confessed to being weak and dizzy. I didn't know the cause of the diarrhea, but I knew he needed to go straight to the hospital where his lost fluids and electrolytes could be replaced.

There was a laboratory technician at the hospital who I admired for her ability to find parasites and their ova, so I asked her to take a look at my patient's stool sample. With such work you have to be patient and thorough as sometimes there may only be a few parasites in a sample. It wasn't long before this technician gave me a call, saying, "Your patient's stool specimen is loaded with giardia parasites and cysts."

This man had giardiasis, a parasitic infection of the small bowel by a single-celled organism called *Giardia lamblia*. It's also called beaver fever since beavers often carry the parasite and contaminate streams and lakes with the cysts. That's why campers and hikers are encouraged to boil their drinking water. I was familiar with giardiasis because my sister Jewel and her family worked at a mission school along the Amazon River in Brazil, and I always checked the whole family when they returned on furlough for parasites. One of my young nieces once had a few cysts of *Giardia lamblia* in her stool, but I had never before come across a patient in my practice who had them.

I quizzed this man about whether he had taken any overseas trips or visits to areas in this country where he might have consumed contaminated water. When he said, "no," I asked his wife to bring in some water from their well to be tested, but the sample was negative. I did learn that the patient had sold his pigs several weeks earlier before getting sick. Now he had no animals, except for his dog and a runt pig that was too small to sell with the others. I called our local veterinarian and asked him to check out the runt pig. Dr. Reed reported back that the pig was loaded with giardia.

But then the question was how did my patient get the disease from his pigs? That was answered when I learned that he had used hog manure on his garden that spring. In fact, because of that fertilizer, his garden produced a tremendous crop of vegetables—the best yield ever. We checked the stool of the other family members, but they were negative. His wife said she always cleaned the vegetables well before using them, even the ones she bought in the store. My patient evidently acquired the parasite on his hands while working in the garden. The mystery was solved, and he soon returned to work.

Earlier in my practice I had another parasitic mystery. This one involved a farmer who lived about five miles from Markle. He had been a farmer all of his adult life, and now that his children were married, he and his wife lived alone on the farm. One autumn he became sick but figured he only had the flu since he ran a low-grade fever with some diarrhea, nausea, and weight loss. After about a week of these symptoms, he started getting abdominal pain associated with the diarrhea and also a higher fever.

When he came to the office, I sent him immediately to the hospital. This was in the mid-60s when the only studies we could do of the intestines were barium swallows and enemas. After the radiologist performed the barium enema, he said my patient had amoebiasis. The only time he had ever seen anything like this was in Vietnam, when he was an army radiologist. When I called the hospital laboratory, the technician confirmed the presence of *Entamoeba histolytica* in his stool specimen. The radiologist felt that there were multiple infected abscesses in the patient's intestines but said there was no effective treatment for the disease. The ill farmer received all the recommended treatment that was then available, but his high fever persisted and he slipped into a coma.

Where did someone in Markle pick up amoebiasis? There were no other known patients with amoebic dysentery in the surrounding areas, and I had never seen it even in medical school. Although not common in Indiana, this disease is widely spread throughout the world—especially in the tropics. The one-celled *Entamoeba histolytica* is found only in humans and is carried in human excrement. It is most common in Asia where farmers are more apt to use human feces as fertilizer on gardens and fields.

Sir Arthur Conan Doyle wrote, "When you have eliminated all which is impossible, then whatever remains, however improbable, must be the truth." My patient's wife said that in the past twenty years her husband had not been anywhere except at home and in the surrounding four counties. I talked to our local health department, and it agreed to canvas the community to see if there had been any unusual happenings. The investigation discovered that an injured Vietnam soldier had come home to stay with his parents, just before my patient became ill. That family lived about a half mile away, and the parents said their son had been treated for some parasite they thought was amoeba. My patient had not visited them, but a small stream ran past both homes. I thought we had solved the mystery, but we could not verify all of the facts and I couldn't help wondering why this farmer developed the disease's worst complications. It was only one or two years later that the effective drug Flagyl (metronidazole) was developed, but by then it was far too late for my patient who died about a month after falling into the coma.

Sometimes when I tried to solve a medical mystery I felt like I was grasping at straws. In the early 90s, Steve Binkley, a counselor and administrator at our office, asked me if I would assume care of his mother-in-law who had just been placed in a local nursing home. Steve's wife told me that her mother had been fine until several weeks earlier when she started becoming confused, weak, and unable to care for herself. Char had brought her from Ohio to Lutheran Hospital where she had undergone multiple tests but continued to deteriorate. As a last resort the neurosurgeon performed an open biopsy of her brain which showed no specific disease, only inflammation. The patient had become minimally communicative and the neurosurgeon as well as other physicians felt there was nothing more they could do to help her.

When I first saw my patient in the nursing home, it did appear that she was not going to live much longer. But I reasoned that since the biopsy showed inflammation we should at least treat her for that and see what might happen. If we didn't see any improvement, we would discontinue the therapy.

Within only a few days, this woman started regaining her strength, and by the next week I could converse much better with her. During the next month, she continued to improve and soon was walking. After a few more months, she was begging to go home. She went on to live another fifteen years after her near-death experience, with no residual effects. I never knew what caused the inflammation, possibly a virus she had recovered from or some toxic agent.

Diagnosis can be difficult when symptoms mimic those of a more common disease. At first a seventy-five-year-old patient's memory loss seemed to be the onset of Alzheimer's disease. He had lived his entire life in Markle but had seldom come into the office. His wife approached me one day, saying, "I'm no longer able to look after my husband. He's confused. He wanders off and forgets what happened yesterday." When I saw him, he appeared alert but only spoke when I asked him questions—and his answers were only one or two words. His tone of voice was flat, and I could not get him to smile. He didn't know the day of the week or what he had done the day before, but he did know his name and who I was. He could answer questions about his childhood and early years of marriage yet scored toward the severe category when I gave him several mental status tests to determine the degree of impairment from dementia.

His wife insisted that he needed to be placed in a nursing home so that she could get some rest. I made arrangements for his admission and over the next several months was able to observe him closely. He posed no problems for the staff; he easily let the nurses and aides care for him. I usually found him sitting in a chair with his Cubs baseball cap on. He'd ask me the same two questions over and over again: "When am I going to eat?" and "Are the Cubs playing today?" I discovered that he was actually very knowledgeable about Cub history and the stats of some of the old-time players.

As months passed, I saw no further deterioration of his mental functions. This was odd for Alzheimer's. I started questioning my diagnosis. In talking with his wife and friends, I discovered that this patient had a history of high alcohol intake. While he was still working, he drank moderately during the week and heavily on weekends. But once he retired, he drank very heavily each day and ate poorly. In the late nineteenth century, Sergei Korsakoff, a

Russian neuropsychiatrist, described a condition of dementia in alcoholics in which they had retrograde amnesia and an apathetic attitude. The disorder, now called Korsakoff's syndrome, is actually caused by a lack of thiamine (Vitamin B1), but that deficiency is usually linked to chronic alcohol abuse. Alcohol interferes with the conversion of thiamine to the active form of the vitamin, and it often inflames the stomach lining so that frequent vomiting affects the absorption of B1. Heavy drinkers often have poor diets, as well, and this limits their vitamin intake.

Korsakoff's syndrome caused my patient to lose a vital sense of connection to much of his life, and he remained fixated on his remote past when he was keenly interested in the Cubs baseball team. Even though he was in the nursing home for months without any alcoholic drinks, his mental condition did not improve. The brain damage was permanent.

I'm reminded of another patient who I admitted to a local nursing home with the initial diagnosis of Alzheimer's. This man was in his late seventies, and the course of his disease was rather rapid. He had a loss of memory for recent events and appeared depressed, with a flat, dull affect. His wife had passed away about a year before, and this had changed his life greatly as they were always together after his retirement. His children were supportive and helpful, but they were getting frustrated with his inability to do anything for himself. They thought that if he was in a different environment and could talk to individuals his own age he might improve.

But during the first months at the retirement center, his condition continued to decline. In fact, the deterioration was rapid even for a patient with Alzheimer's. When I gave him physical examinations, everything seemed normal except that he had poor balance. He hadn't had any falls that we knew of, but the examination indicated he was at risk.

We decided to move this man to an area of the center where he would receive more care. But before moving him, I ordered a CAT scan of his brain. The results surprised us by revealing that he had increased intracranial pressure due to an abnormal accumulation of cerebrospinal fluid in the ventricles of the brain. Though very rare, this condition, known as normal pressure hydrocephalus, is one that needs to be ruled out in patients with dementia. We have had several older patients over the years with this problem, but they've all been diagnosed after falling. A neurosurgeon implanted a ventriculoperitoneal shunt to drain excess cerebrospinal fluid to the abdomen where it was harmlessly absorbed. His depression improved after that, and gradually he regained his mental abilities. He moved into an independent living apartment and even enjoyed going on trips with his family.

One time I was called on a morning house call to a family whose chief complaint was that they were having chronic headaches. The husband and wife were in their mid-70s and cared for their adult daughter who had cerebral palsy. The wife told me that she thought her husband was also occasionally mildly confused. From my examinations nothing appeared out of the ordinary, and at the time they said their headaches were a bit better. I suggested that they come into the office for lab work, but all the lab results were normal.

I thought the family was probably going to be okay, but a week later I received a call saying that they all had terrible headaches and didn't feel they could even safely drive to the office. I again made a house call and discovered that they had no fever, their blood pressures were normal, and nothing seemed unusual other than their headaches. By the end of the visit, they told me that they were again feeling better. Then I thought of the car mechanic I had recently seen in the office. He worked in a vented garage but late in the afternoon was getting headaches that made him leave work. I had taken a carbon monoxide level on him and discovered it to be very high. When the ventilation in the garage was improved, the headaches disappeared.

With that case in mind I had a nurse from the Wells County Health Department come to the home and draw blood samples. They showed elevated carbon monoxide levels in all three of the family members. A new furnace had recently been installed so I told them that since it was spring and the weather had turned warm, they should switch off the furnace and have it inspected for leaks. The man who installed the furnace came to the house and told them the heater was fine. But later that spring, when the weather turned colder, the family turned the furnace back on and again came down with headaches. They said it couldn't be the furnace because the furnace man said everything was okay.

I told them I was going to get to the bottom of the problem by having all three family members admitted to the hospital. Once there, they all got better. I called the gas company, and after taking a look, the inspector said there was a gas leak and that the furnace had been improperly installed. After someone fixed the problem, there were no more headaches, but I noticed that neither parent ever seemed to be quite as alert as before the poisoning. Since their failing memories did not progress into the usual symptoms of Alzheimer's disease, I feel that some of that memory loss was from chronic exposure to carbon monoxide.

In a sense, every patient with a problem brings a mystery to be solved. I suppose that's one of the many reasons I enjoyed my medical practice so much. The detective in me liked tracking down the root cause of an illness or condition. Sometimes this would involve working with lab technicians and specialists and took days or weeks. But sometimes the mystery only took minutes with no more equipment than a stethoscope.

Such was the case I solved after helping a middle-aged couple to lose weight. This couple had been childless but with the adoption of their son became concerned about their health and motivated to lose weight. I placed them on a diet plan that I used for diabetics, and they came in weekly to be weighed on our scales. In a year the wife lost a hundred pounds and the husband lost sixty. They were both pleased and said they had never felt so well.

Several months later, however, the wife made an appointment to see me. She was extremely anxious and told my nurse, "I have a tumor in my stomach, and I'm afraid it's cancer. Now after finally losing all that weight, I'm going to die."

I examined her stomach and felt the large mass. I told her that the mass was moving and that it had a heartbeat. She was about full term but hadn't guessed she was pregnant because she hadn't experienced a menstrual period for many years, something not uncommon in an overweight woman.

She and her husband were excited and pleased when a healthy, eight-pound baby was delivered three weeks later.

OFFICE PSYCHOLOGY

In addition to having detective skills, a good doctor needs to understand human psychology.

My predecessor Dr. Woods had insight into that area. He saw a link between a pill's color and its perceived efficacy, a connection that scientists have only recently discovered. In a 2010 issue of the *International Journal of Biotechnology*, R. K. Srivastava and colleagues report that the color of a pill can boost its placebo effect. Red and pink tablets, they assert, are favored over other shades.

Dr. Wood's medicines were still on the pharmacy shelves when we moved in. We noticed that he had stocked three colors of five grain aspirin: pink, white, and orange — all the same size and cost. We continued to stock these three colors because some patients would tell us, "Those pink pills really work great. Give me more of those." Or another patient would say, "Only the orange pills give me relief, but my wife finds that the pink ones work best for her pain." Hardly any patients asked for the white pills. Aspirin is an old drug that can be helpful not just for the treatment of pain but also to help prevent heart attacks, blood clots, and inflammation. Fifty years ago when there were very few safe pain medications, Dr. Woods discovered a way to get the most positive results from an inexpensive medicine that was effectual and safe.

When Lee and I took over his office, I felt it lacked the nice, clean, medicinal smell that I associate with such places — maybe because it had stood unused for a year. After a while, I discovered that squirting a few drops of Camoral on the counter would give us that fragrance I missed. I had never heard of this injectable medicine before, but it supposedly helped colds. We never felt it helped to shorten any of the symptoms so we didn't recommend it to patients. However, I kept a bottle in the office for many years, just to freshen the air and cover the scent of popcorn when patients complained that the place smelled more like a theatre than a doctor's office. Some of the nurses still accuse me of shooting Camoral from a syringe and leaving yellow stains on the white ceiling tiles. This recklessness escapes my recollection, but if such was the case, the psychological effect was worth it. Scientists will undoubtedly discover one day that the odor of a doctor's office is as significant to patients as the color and size of their pills.

Before the use of ultrasounds to check the progression of pregnancies, parents would not know the sex of their child until the infant was laid on the mother's stomach after delivery. Doctors often told mothers that if the fetus's heart rate was over 140 the child would be a girl and if less than 140, a boy. That rule of thumb was accurate about fifty percent of the time. During my first years at Markle, local mothers felt that they had a better way to predict the sex of their child. At this time we kept a tablet in the office that listed all of our deliveries, with the date, doctor, and gender. Lee and I delivered about the same number of babies, but for a few years the percentage of males and females we delivered was very lop-sided. Word got out, and community women started saying that if Lee delivered their baby it would be a boy and if I did, it would be a girl.

This pattern held true—or mostly true—for a few years, and then mothers once again wanted me to predict the sex of their child. I found a more effective way to handle gender questions then the old heart rate method. When a mother asked me what the sex of her baby would be, I asked whether she wanted a son or a daughter. Then I would tell her she was having the opposite. Or if she already had three or more of one sex, I told her she would have another of the same sex. If the baby turned out to be what I predicted, the mother was content because we had known all along the child's gender. If my prediction was wrong, she was so happy that I was wrong that she didn't care what I had told her. I could not lose either way.

In the 60s and 70s, many doctors still felt, "What patients don't know won't hurt them." Maybe in 1854 during the Crimean War when the poet Alfred Lord Tennyson wrote "The Charge of the Light Brigade" it was appropriate to say of soldiers, "Theirs not to reason why, theirs but to do and die," but I don't consider it a proper attitude to take toward patients. I've always felt that they need to be partners in the dialogue and cure. They need to understand their diseases and the reasons behind their treatments. I have felt this so strongly that I often told my patients more than they needed or even wanted to know. Patients will forget much of what they hear from a doctor, but if I repeated the same information in different ways and provided print-outs, they would retain some of the knowledge.

I observed that the psychological impact of education on a patient could be dramatic at any age. For a while I was educating the mother of a twelve-year-old girl who had juvenile diabetes about her daughter's disease, but when the diabetes remained difficult to manage, I decided I was focusing on the wrong person. After I turned my attention to educating the young patient, she started to gain control over her disease.

Sometimes I was tempted to dismiss some of my patients as hypochondriacs, but I learned that I should always listen closely to their symptoms and approach the illness as if they really had a problem. Some people were so convinced they were ill that it was better to find something to treat than to tell them they needed no treatment. If I just dismissed their problem as insignificant, they might go to another practitioner whose treatment might actually be harmful. It was also important for me to pay attention and not jump to a hasty judgment because there just might really be an underlying medical problem.

For instance, when one of my older patients who often came in for insignificant problems complained of severe stomach pains, I had her abdomen x-rayed at the hospital. We discovered she had a distended stomach where a trichobezoar (hairball) was lodged. I had noticed that her hair was getting thinner but hadn't suspected that she was pulling it out and swallowing it.

In the x-ray I had noticed that dozens of undigested pills were caught in the hairball, so after it was dissolved and my patient was released from the hospital, I visited her at home. By her bed was a large glass candy dish in which she had poured all of her pills whenever she received a new prescription. All those colors and sizes of pills mixed together certainly did make an attractive design. She said she knew what each pill was for, but when I quizzed her, she made many mistakes.

I confiscated everything in the candy dish and told her we would start over again, with only the pills she needed.

HUMOR IN THE OFFICE

Folks in Markle enjoy a good joke. But you would expect that from a town that boasts on its entry sign: "Home of 1,102 Happy People and 4 grouches." During the Depression, a town joke club met in the bakery's basement. To join this club you had to do something ridiculous. For instance, Jay Hayes wore a coon-skin coat for two weeks in the summer.

The pranksters who once pulled an elaborate joke on Wade Randol, the town barber, were probably charter members of this club. When they heard that Wade was ordering an expensive coon dog from down south, they intercepted the dog along the train route and swapped it for an old stray. Wade's son Bob recalls what happened after the Markle stationmaster called to say his father's dog had arrived: "Father's friends went with him and shook their heads. They told him, 'You really got took.'" Since Wade was an accomplished prankster, these friends might have orchestrated the joke as a payback. "All that dog would do was chase cats," Bob said. The joke went on for a week, until his father's friends finally gave him the right dog.

The doctors and nurses at the Markle Medical Center had some prankster tendencies, too. It took me a couple of years, but eventually I realized that on April Fools' Day I should refrain from any of the sweets that Janice Jordan, our LPN, brought to the office. What looked like chocolate-covered cherries were chocolate-covered cotton balls. Crème puffs appeared harmless, but inside they harbored more wads of cotton. During the rest of the year, Janice's baked goods were a real treat since she was an exceptional cook.

The mission statement for the Markle Medical Center asserts that physicians and personnel are to work "in a comfortable and congenial atmosphere." Lee was adept at creating that atmosphere. He was a naturally gregarious man with a quick wit, who brought a sense of humor with him whenever he entered a room. When something went wrong, he could see the comedy or irony of the situation, assisted, no doubt, by the perspective espoused in his favorite saying: "In light of eternity, what does it matter?"

We both believed that humor is a useful prescription for stress and could help break the strain from a long day of appointments or a night busy with urgent house calls. Some of the most humorous experiences I had while seeing patients might have added to the stress if I hadn't seen the humor.

For example, early in my medical practice a sixteen-year-old girl came to see me about losing weight. She was moderately overweight, but by no means obese, and I supposed she was looking for some sort of diet pills although she never really asked for any. Since I seldom prescribed diet medications and certainly never any pills to teenagers, we spent a considerable amount of time discussing her dietary habits and what she could do to help control her weight. She needed to reduce her caloric intake, increase her exercise, and realize that weight loss is a long range goal. We talked about specific changes she could make, and I repeatedly emphasized the importance of willpower.

Then I asked her, "Do you have any willpower?"

She answered, "Grandma buys it once in a while, but I really don't care for it."

I felt I had lost the battle that day.

Another instance of miscommunication grew apparent as I was making a house call one evening in the home of an elderly couple where the husband had been ill with vomiting and an upset stomach for the past twenty-four hours. During the examination, the wife requested, "Don't give my husband any of those suppositories for vomiting because the last time you gave them the edges really hurt him something terrible." I found out that he had never removed the tinfoil from the suppository. After that experience I always wrote on the envelope, "Remove tinfoil before inserting rectally."

Another time I was talking with a patient—a burly farmer—who said, "I need you to straighten out a problem. What's the color of the blood pressure pills that you gave me? I've been taking a yellow pill, but my wife says that's her hormone medicine." I told him that his pills were white and that, yes, he was taking his wife's hormone pills. For months after that, each time I saw this man he would greet me in a falsetto voice.

Much humor is rooted in the absurdity or incongruity of a situation. That was the case many years ago as I sat at the end of an examination table to give a woman with her feet in the stirrups a regular pelvic exam with Pap smear. I couldn't believe my eyes and looked at the nurse who was smiling. There, stuck on the woman's bottom, was an S&H Green Stamp. We controlled ourselves so that the woman would not be embarrassed.

A physical examination can be embarrassing enough just by its nature, but one time I made one worse than it should have been by changing a protocol and not anticipating the results. Our office did a lot of pre-employee physical examinations for local industries, and to save time I told my nurse that she should instruct the men to strip to their shorts before I came in. Soon after we initiated that new instruction, I walked into a room and found a blushing young man seated in the corner, totally in the nude. I hadn't realized that a number of young men did not wear any underwear. I tried not to show my surprise and did a quick hernia check along with the normal physical exam. After that episode we changed our instruction to asking the men to strip to their waist.

Sometimes the humor of a situation wasn't detected until after some detective work cleared up a mystery. For example, a woman in her seventies came to see me one Monday afternoon with a peculiar problem. "Every Sunday for the past month while I sit in church, I've heard a beeping in my ear," she said. "It happens about halfway through the sermon. The worse part of it is that people around me also hear it and look at me. But my husband who's next to me doesn't hear a thing. I'm confused about this and embarrassed." I told her to come to the office the next day at 10:45 a.m.

I entered the room a few minutes before 11 o'clock that Tuesday and started quietly examining her. At exactly on the hour she exclaimed, "There! The beeping is starting again. Can you hear it?" I held her left wrist up to her ear. After she got over her embarrassment, we had a good laugh together. Then I disabled the alarm on her new wristwatch and suggested that her husband have his hearing checked.

Office humor was often mixed with a sense of relief. A few years before I retired, an eighty-eight-year-old woman saw me for a routine appointment. She was a long-time patient who lived by herself now but came to the office accompanied by two of her daughters who worked at the hospital—one as the head nurse and the other as a respiratory therapist. They had recently traveled to Virginia with their mother to visit a sister suffering some medical problems.

"I have something that I haven't told anyone about," my patient said. "I noticed a painful, raised up mole on my back before we went to Virginia, but I didn't tell the girls because I thought they might not let me go and this might be the last trip I ever make to see my daughter. I think this black mole might be what you call a melanoma. You can do whatever you think should be done now that I'm back."

After her daughters helped strip her down to the waist, it was easy to see the problem. She did, in fact, have a sizeable, elevated, black spot on her back. I took a sharp-nosed forceps and removed the largest tick I had ever seen. I showed it to the patient, and we shared a good laugh. This tick had been feeding for at least a month and was well engorged—the size of a dime.

Sometimes the joke was on me. For instance, I'll never forget the day I must have missed a patient's chart or mislaid it. Anyway, when we were finished seeing patients for that day, my nurse Janet Himes started straightening up the rooms. When she entered one examination room, she was startled to see a middle-aged man seated in a chair. With a bemused smile, he said, "I've been sitting here since two o'clock, and it's now five-thirty. I was going to give Dr. Miller another fifteen minutes, and if he didn't show up I was going to leave." Janet ran out to catch me as I was getting in my car. Needless to say, I apologized profusely as I spent time caring for what might have been Markle's most good-humored patient.

Mark Twain once wrote, "The wit knows that his place is at the tail of a procession." That day I felt I belonged with the wit.

REFERRALS

Initially, the referral physicians Lee and I used were ones we observed during our internship and admired for their skills, knowledge, and patient care. Some of these older doctors served as my mentors, counseling me on what procedures I should or should not perform. For instance, one evening I came to the emergency room at Lutheran Hospital with a twelve-year-old girl who had fallen from a tree and appeared to have fractured her left elbow. I ordered an x-ray and called in an orthopedic surgeon. When he saw my patient, he said, "Gerald, this is a fracture you should be treating yourself. I know you've been told in lectures never to treat a supracondylar fracture, but this is one I don't need to see." He then described the fracture, how to apply the cast, and conduct the follow-up. He even suggested how to charge for the care and casting. After speaking with the patient and her parents, this doctor left without charging a penny. Lee and I had numerous mentoring experiences like this one in our early years.

Later the specialists we used included doctors we knew through personal acquaintance or had heard speak at medical meetings. Besides expecting these doctors to know their area of expertise well and to relate well to patients, we expected them to send us a letter in a timely manner so we would know what they were thinking and what kind of treatment they recommended. I particularly appreciated the doctors who would pick up the phone to give me a personal call.

Several conditions would rule out certain specialists for referrals. For instance, we wouldn't send patients to a physician who two or more of our patients didn't like. I remember patients complaining about one oncologist who after checking them over would rub his chin and with a deliberately negative tone, say, "This is bad, very bad. I don't expect a good result, but I will do everything I can for you." He said this even with cancers that had almost a hundred percent cure rate. He may have been covering himself, but it was overly discouraging to patients and their families.

I also ruled out any physicians who were dishonest with patients, like the pediatrician who told an eleven-year-old boy that the cancer in his leg bone was only an infection. He told the parents the truth but told them not to tell their son. They lived with that lie until their son died and always regretted it. In fact, that lie led the family to mistrust all doctors. Several years later when the second son came in with a sore ankle, he became hysterical when I told him it was only a sprain. He remembered how the doctor had lied to his brother and now had a problem trusting me.

Then there was the urologist who phoned both Lee and me one day and said, "If the IRS calls you, I want you to tell them that you used my condominium on Lake Wawasee for a week last summer. Will you do that?" We told him, no; we would not do that. Neither of us had ever gone to his condo. That was the end of using that urologist for referrals. If he wasn't honest with the government, how could we trust him to be honest with us or our patients?

My basic rule of thumb was to never recommend a specialist I wouldn't use for myself or my wife and children. This eliminated the rough-mannered ears-nose-throat specialist who worked on my patient one night at the Lutheran Hospital emergency room; it was clear that he didn't have enough regard for his Hippocratic Oath—to do no harm. The night before, this patient had developed a severe posterior nosebleed that I treated with a catheter. After extending the tube through the nose, I filled the balloon with water, pulled it into a tight position, and secured it with an anterior nasal pack. I usually left such catheters in place for three days, but the next evening, my patient called, saying the catheter was uncomfortable and since he wasn't having any more bleeding, he wanted it removed. Against my better judgment, I removed the packing and the catheter. Immediately, the nose started bleeding heavily. I told the patient he would need to go to the hospital emergency room, and I offered to drive him myself since his wife who was at home with two young children was also pregnant and near term.

The ears-nose-throat specialist on call said he would have to repack the nose and admit the patient to the hospital. As he roughly pushed and shoved, the patient cried out in terrible anguish, worse than anything I had ever heard. The surgeon just scolded him, saying such things as "Shut up. You're a baby. You're a wimp. What's wrong with you? Can't you stand a little pain?" This doctor berated the man the whole time he worked on his bleeding nose. He never gave him any pain medicine, either.

The next morning when I returned for hospital rounds, I saw that the left side of my patient's face was black and blue and swollen. I ordered an x-ray of the facial bones that revealed a fracture of the left maxillary bone. This was the reason the patient had such severe pain—the doctor had broken his cheekbone. Soon after this experience I was relieved to learn that this physician was dismissed from the group practice he founded.

MONITORING DOCTORS

When I was an intern at Lutheran, hospitals and medical societies had not yet joined to monitor the ethics and skills of the medical community. Sometimes intoxicated physicians arrived at the hospital to deliver a baby or respond to an emergency. Other doctors tried to cover for them, but little was done to control the problem by taking punitive measures.

At Wells Community Hospital we did not have a problem with doctors under the influence of alcohol or other drugs, but sometimes as these doctors aged they didn't realize that their physical skills were impaired. In these instances we had the difficult task of telling these experienced physicians to stop performing certain surgeries. One physician had to be told he couldn't assist with surgeries because he had started passing out during them. I had to inform another that neither Lee nor I would give any anesthesia for his surgeries because his hands were too uncoordinated and shaky.

"Young fellow," the doctor snapped, "I have performed more surgeries than you have or ever will. I know when I should quit. Don't ever tell me what I can or cannot do."

A few days later, though, he came up to me and apologized. Over a cup of coffee he thanked me for caring about him and helping him to confront his limitations. We stayed good friends until he died a few years later.

We had a more difficult problem at the hospital when one of the physician groups hired a new surgeon to join their practice. This doctor had been working in an Illinois city, but now wanted to practice in a rural area. He brought letters of recommendation with him, and the hospital gave him surgical privileges.

Assisted by some of the general practitioners in his group, this doctor started out doing some minor surgeries, including such abdominal procedures as hysterectomies, appendectomies, and gall bladder removals. When I gave the anesthesia for some of these, it was evident to me that the surgeon was counting on his associates for directions. Several of his techniques appeared dangerous, but when I questioned him, he'd say, "Oh, that's just a new method I've learned. Don't worry. It'll be okay."

On his third week he was scheduled to perform a vaginal hysterectomy and I was to give the anesthetic. No one assisting had ever performed this type of hysterectomy; we had always brought in a surgeon from Fort Wayne or sent the patient to Lutheran. After I put the patient to sleep, the new surgeon came in and sat down at the end of the operating table. He made a few cuts and then just sat there. I said, "What's wrong?"

He poked around a little and then answered, "I can't go ahead right now. I'm sick. I need to lie down." He looked pale and was sweating profusely.

When he left, I asked the assistant, his associate, "What do we do now?" He said to give the doctor a few minutes since he was sure he'd return.

In about ten minutes he did come back, re-scrubbed and ready to go. He sat down again, made one more incision, and then stood up, saying, "I'm too sick to continue. I'll need to leave."

Since the surgery had already started, we decided that the assistant would go ahead and do an abdominal hysterectomy, a procedure he was very capable of performing. He finished and everything went well.

Afterwards I advised the hospital administrator to check this surgeon's credentials. We discovered that he was, indeed, a physician with a valid Indiana license. However, he wasn't a licensed surgeon. In Illinois he had worked in an out-patient hospital, assisting a surgeon. From just watching, he decided that surgery was easy and that he could do it himself.

After that, the hospital carefully verified all medical credentials, following the precept of the poet John Donne who wrote, "I observe the physician with the same diligence as the disease."

SIX: GROUP PRACTICE

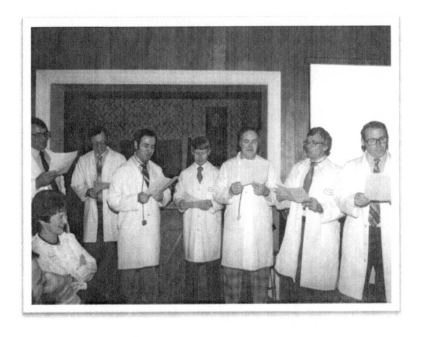

VIC

Six years after moving to Markle, I received a phone call from Rose Lampton, a patient seeing us for maternity care. She said, "My brother, Victor Binkley, is finishing his surgical residency in Hawaii and looking for a place to go into practice. He's flying in and borrowing our car to visit some groups in the East that have been recruiting him. But I told him about your practice, and he's interested in talking with you. I was hoping you'd meet with him and show him around."

Lee and I had never considered adding another doctor to our practice, let alone a surgeon, but we agreed to meet with Rose's brother and to show him our office. We spent about three hours together, describing our work in the community and our philosophy of medical practice. Dr. Binkley told us that he grew up in Northeastern Illinois and graduated from Ohio State Medical School. After his internship, he'd been drafted and served two years as a medical Captain in the Army—one year in Vietnam and the other in El Paso, Texas. Lee and I were impressed with his medical credentials and his articulate responses to our questions, but we questioned whether there were enough surgical needs in the area to support a surgeon.

Two days after Dr. Binkley had left to visit the doctors recruiting him, he called to say, "I've been to a couple of the places on my list, but all I can think about is Markle. I'd like to cancel the rest of my trip and spend the last day or two before I have to go back to Hawaii observing your practice."

Lee and I were surprised by this turn of events, but we liked Victor and the idea that with a third doctor we'd only need to be on call every third weekend. Another doctor would also help us stay better apprised of new medical advances since we could more easily take turns going to post-graduate courses. But would a surgeon be a good fit for our practice? Could we afford to add one?

When Victor came back, he let us know that he loved surgery but that he also enjoyed other aspects of medicine, including pediatric and obstetrical care. When we told him we shared call and the same salaries, but that we were open to other possibilities, he said our arrangements were just fine. He wasn't concerned about his salary; he was more interested in giving good care to his patients and being in a practice in which the doctors got along. Victor flew back to Hawaii and then sent us word that his wife, Carol, felt positive about coming to Markle. Within two weeks everything was agreed upon and Victor started the process of getting his Indiana medical license.

We soon discovered that Vic was someone who thought outside of the box. He made helpful suggestions on practical things like record keeping and improving the flow of patients through the office. "Work smart, not hard," was one of his favorite sayings.

By the first week, Lee and I were also aware of Vic's impressive surgical skills as he performed the hernia repairs and minor surgeries we had reserved for him. During the second week I called Vic to the hospital to see a patient being admitted in critical condition; this man was cold and clammy, with a weak, thready pulse. He obviously had massive internal bleeding from a stomach ulcer, and I asked Vic to come from the office as quickly as possible. Meanwhile, I gave the patient blood to keep his pressure up, but I could see we were losing him. Normally, this was a patient I would have promptly sent to the Fort Wayne hospital but with the concern that he might die en route.

Vic assessed the patient's condition and said he needed surgery immediately. I asked him if he could do the surgery. "I know that I can do it," said Vic, "but the question is, are you confident that I can?"

I had never seen anyone perform a stomach resection so quickly and smoothly. The patient had a successful recovery and was soon back selling investments.

Vic was the first surgeon in the area to do same day discharge for hernia repairs. He said, "If patients can go to Toronto and get same day discharge, they can come to Wells Community Hospital and go home the same day." He also decided that there was no good reason why patients after gall bladder surgery needed tubes in their stomach. Over the years, he easily kept up with new surgical advances and became adept at endoscopic and laparoscopic procedures.

In fact, Vic was always learning new things about all of his varied interests: horticulture, landscaping, carpentry, history, literature, politics, religion, stained-glass art, birds. The list was extensive. We thought maybe Vic knew everything, until the day he accidently injured his favorite cat with the lawnmower and decided he could treat her himself. Before stitching up her side, he gave her a shot of Demerol.

Instead of helping her to relax, that injection turned his patient into a hyperactive wildcat. When he finally got her to the vet, Dr. Reed let Vic know what he had already deduced—that when it comes to felines, Demerol changes

Dr. Jekyll into Mr. Hyde. "You're a good surgeon for humans," Doc Reed told him, "but stay away from cats."

THE HORN OF AFRICA

About a year after Vic had joined our practice, he asked Lee and me if we had ever considered overseas mission work. We admitted that we had but thought we could never leave the remaining doctor or doctors with so much to do.

"With an attitude like that, you will never feel like you can go overseas," Vic said. "Now that there are three doctors here, we should be able to get away on a rotating basis. While one doctor is gone, the other two can be financially supporting him and carrying on the practice." Lee and I agreed that the idea was feasible. We would pray about it and talk with our wives.

Soon we had a more formal discussion and everyone was in accord. If the circumstances arose for overseas medical work, one of us could go for up to a year, with partial economic support from the two doctors in Markle.

Mary and I were surprised several weeks later when we received a letter from Eastern Mennonite Mission Board in Salunga, Pennsylvania, asking if I would serve a year at Shirati Hospital in Tanzania. One of the hospital's doctors had just left, and another doctor was needed soon. This was March of 1971, and the mission board wanted a doctor no later than that upcoming July. Mary was less enthusiastic about the opportunity than I, but Shari, Marlis, and Steve saw it as an appealing adventure.

In May as we were in the midst of making decisions about what we would do about our house for a year and where Shari and Marlis would go to school, the mission board contacted us again, asking if we would consider changing our assignment from Tanzania to Somalia. The village of Jamama needed an emergency fill-in doctor for a year to serve as the only doctor at the Mennonite hospital, clinic, and nursing school. The board had trouble justifying another doctor to the Shirati staff while there were no doctors at all in Jamama. It felt I would be well-suited since I was a general practitioner trained in obstetrics, surgery, and medicine.

Since we would be in Somalia for only a year, the mission board said we wouldn't need to take language study or the usual classes in cultural orientation. But we wanted to know something about Somalia, so we pulled out our *World Book Encyclopedia*. What we learned about our new destination seemed to resonate with what Mrs. Gibbs says in Thornton Wilder's *Our Town*: "Only it seems to me that once in your life before you die you ought to see a country where they don't talk in English and don't even want to."

Somalia fit the bill. It was on the Horn of Africa, 99.9 percent Muslim, and much of it desert inhabited by nomads. The village of Jamama was in the southern part of the country, in an agricultural district where farmers irrigated their fields from the Juba River. It was probably best that we didn't know too much about the country before we left— especially its political situation—or we might not have had the nerve to leave home.

When my patients heard that I would be gone for a year, most offered me encouragement, though some said, "Why would you go to a foreign country, when you're needed right here?" I explained that the Jamama hospital was in desperate need of a doctor and that I would be the only physician for thirty miles. In Somalia, the second poorest country in the world, even seriously ill or injured patients often had to walk to see the doctor, a journey that could take several days or more. Our church family at the Markle Church of the Brethren already had an interest in supporting overseas service. They never questioned our decision, but gave Mary and me their unreserved support.

When we arrived at Jamama, I noticed how different the village was from Markle. Mud daub or cement houses lined dirt streets and against the sky stood a minaret, rather than a Methodist steeple. But now, forty years later, I'm struck by the similarities. Both were small towns surrounded by agricultural areas and near the banks of an important river. Both were populated by religious people who had lived in the area for generations and who welcomed my family with hospitality and kindness. The Jamama clinic and hospital kept me as busy as their counterparts at home, and my work in all of these locations was so much easier because I had the assistance of excellent nurses and staff.

Shari and I wrote about my Somali experiences in our book, *A Hundred Camels: A Mission Doctor's Sojourn and Murder Trial in Somalia* (Cascadia Publishing House, 2009). This memoir documents my year in Jamama—an immensely rewarding time, despite the stress of being tried for murder when one of my patients died.

While we were gone, nurses at the office rotated writing to us and friends sent many letters, some even weekly, keeping us well-informed of community news. Some patients and friends mailed packages with dry food items, like Jell-O and cake mixes. Because mail service was so slow, we received some packages not long before it was time to leave. One box of cereal left the United States by ship, and when it arrived half a year later, the box was badly torn and the cereal, stale. Still, we deeply valued the thoughtfulness of the sender. After our first six months, Mary wrote an article for *The Bluffton News Banner* describing Somali culture, our daily home life, and my work at the hospital. "There are many snake bites, scorpion bites and recently [Gerald] had one patient who was stepped on by an elephant and another who was picked up and thrown by one," she wrote. That piece stimulated more people to write to us.

Although it was hard leaving our Somali friends and the other mission workers, Mary and I were eager after a year abroad to return to the Markle community. We missed our friends and even the humid Indiana summers that we now viewed as temperate. Jamama was only a few miles from the equator and not much above sea level. The constant desert heat was hard to deal with, especially for Mary. Whereas the rest of us would sweat when we were hot, she would only get over-heated and red. As we planned our return itinerary, a country close to the Arctic Circle seemed enticing, so we spent several days in Bergen, Norway where even in August we could pull on thick woolen sweaters.

We were supposed to arrive at the Fort Wayne airport at 6:00 p.m., but our plane needed mechanical repairs in Oslo and left four hours late. As a result, when we landed at Kennedy Airport, our scheduled flight had left. The airlines offered to put us up overnight in a hotel, but we were so eager to get home that we decided to scramble to catch a flight from LaGuardia. We jumped into a taxi and ran with our suitcases through the terminal to board the plane just as it was ready to leave dock. Then, just as we were beginning to relax in our seats, we passed through a severe storm that tossed our plane, rattled the overhead luggage, and made us wonder whether we were meant to reach home that night.

Near the stroke of midnight, we finally descended toward the Baer Field Airport in Fort Wayne. By that hour we were groggy, and when we touched down, we assumed some celebrity must be onboard because a large crowd was gathered at the outdoor gate, waving hands and hoisting a banner. From inside the plane, we couldn't recognize faces. We didn't know that the welcome was for us until we disembarked and started walking closer. Some of the townspeople had been waiting at the airport since six o'clock and some had driven home and returned to be there when we arrived. We felt blessed to be part of such a caring community.

Over the next few years, doctors from Markle continued on mission trips with their respective churches. Vic served the next year under the Church of God in Bangladesh. By this time Neil Irick had joined our practice as a family physician. We missed our surgeon, but we now had Neil to help with office and hospital visits and go on night calls. When Vic and his family returned from Bangladesh, Lee arranged for a three-month service trip to Zaire with the Methodist Church.

The mid-70s were a time of excitement as we built a larger office at the top of the Markle hill and shared our overseas stories with each other and our community.

PIERRE PAYEN

My cross-cultural experiences didn't end when I returned from Somalia. Four years later the Church of God mission board in Findley, Ohio contacted our office to see if we would partner with them in a new Haitian project. Vic had worked with this mission board in 1974, when he had taken time off from Markle to establish a surgical ward in Bogra, Bangladesh. Since the 1960s, the Church of God mission board had been developing schools, churches, agricultural projects, and nutritional centers in Haiti, and now they wanted to expand to help meet the country's medical needs.

As the poorest country in the Western Hemisphere, Haiti was clearly in need of more medical care. There was a high infant mortality rate and incidence of tuberculosis. Malaria and many of the same tropical diseases we treated in Africa or Bangladesh were present. Our experience in other mission clinics would help us, not only in treating these diseases, but also in setting up a new clinic. At this point, there were five doctors in Markle—David Brown and Joe Greene had joined our practice—and they all agreed that they were interested in this exciting project. With Haiti so close to the United States, travel expenses would be relatively low and we could fly there frequently.

Vic traveled with the mission board chairperson to ascertain the medical needs at Pierre Payen. This village was fifty miles from Port-au-Prince, along the only paved road going north from that city. Although the town was small, farmers walked down from the mountains to sell their produce at the busy open market. Haitians throughout the area came to Pierre Payen to board lorries or brightly painted buses called *tap taps*. The Church of God already had a presence in the community—with a nutritional center, elementary school, and vibrant church.

When he came back, Vic told us the need for medical care in Pierre Payen was great. There were no clinics to serve the dense population surrounding the village and the people in the mountains who came there to trade. Our medical group felt that we could serve the people at Pierre Payen and still provide good care to our patients in the Markle, Bluffton, and Warren areas. The mission board would provide nurses and an administrator for the clinic, and we would supply a physician in blocks of six to eight weeks, with a Haitian doctor from Saint-Marc coming several days each week to help out.

When the clinic opened in the summer of 1977, I was at the dedication ceremony, on my first tour of duty. The day was sweltering, and since government personnel and village leaders spoke for hours and only in Creole, it also seemed lengthy. But I could tell from the smiles and enthusiastic clapping how proud the people were to have a medical facility in their community. And the overall friendliness of the Haitian people was striking. On that trip I learned to appreciate the Haitian proverb: *"Bonjoy se paspo` ou."* "Hello is your passport."

As I did in Somalia, I soon picked up some common words and phrases that were useful in the clinic. I always had a Haitian interpreter, but I usually needed to give the translator some training. A patient might go into great detail describing what was bothering her, and then the new interpreter would say, "She says she has a cough." I'd ask what else the patient said. "Oh, she's just saying some foolish thing about how she got the cough, but it means nothing. It's not worth mentioning." If I pushed for details, the interpreter might say how the patient had two periods last month that gave her the cough or that the cough was due to a cat that crossed her path the previous week. I would need to train my interpreter to always ask right away how long the patient had been sick and what the specific symptoms were.

I quickly ascertained that the number one deadly illness in Haiti was tuberculosis. I might detect it in an elderly, emaciated man who was coughing up blood or in a teenager with a draining infection from a lymph node in her neck. Some of the patients knew they had tuberculosis but wanted to ignore it or maybe they had taken medicine previously but had quit before they were cured.

Usually Haitians with tuberculosis were stoic. When I told them their medical diagnosis, they'd ask only a few questions and show little emotion. However, I will always remember one young mother who had been coughing for six months when she came to see me. When her sputum specimen tested positive for tuberculosis, she started uncontrollably sobbing. "I'm not scared of dying," she said, "but I have a six-month-old daughter and I know that if I die, she will also die."

I explained that if she took her medicine regularly until we told her to quit, she wouldn't die—she would be cured. Over the next two years I saw her many times. Though she lived in a remote area of the mountains, she regularly walked down to get her medicine, sometimes bringing small presents with her, such as a jar of homemade jelly. She always had a pleasant smile, but on the day I could tell her she was cured, it was radiant.

Many of the illnesses I treated in Haiti were similar to those I encountered in Somalia. I saw patients suffering from parasites, tuberculosis, leprosy, malaria, and malnutrition. But, of course, the cultures were different, some of the treatments had changed, and there were illnesses like infantile tetanus, and later AIDS, that I had never treated. During my first visits to Haiti, a number of infants came in with fever and seizures. These newborns had tetanus, and it was heart-rending to watch them die and see the grief on their parents' faces. In Haiti, where virtually all babies are delivered at home by older women serving as midwives, the traditional practice dictates that after the baby is delivered, the cord is cut, usually with a rusty razor blade, and the end of the umbilical cord is dipped in cow dung. The mid-wives didn't detect the connection because not every baby contracts tetanus by this procedure. Our clinic, however, was seeing about one baby a week with tetanus until we started free prenatal classes for the women and gave each one a tetanus shot and a kit supplied by U.S. churches, consisting of a blanket, gown, soap, safety pins, a short piece of umbilical tape to tie the cord, and a new razor blade. Such efforts were initiated all over Haiti by missions and government groups. Today it is rare to see a child with infant tetanus unless that child was born in a remote mountain village.

Haiti seems to have more than its fair share of disasters, and each one contributes to the country's poverty. For instance, soon after we opened the clinic, the Swine Fever Virus was discovered in some of the pigs. Hogs were a principal source of income for many Haitians, but every pig in the country had to be slaughtered. In 1983 we started seeing some very sick young men from Port-au-Prince who showed signs of an illness we had not seen before. Then in 1985 it was learned and widely publicized that AIDS was present in Haiti. Fear of that disease, as well as political unrest, caused the shut-down of the tourism industry which had been developing along the coast.

When Haiti's dictator, Baby Doc, was overthrown in 1986, Joe Greene was working at the clinic. No one knew how the new regime would treat foreigners, but it worried us that all air flights were cancelled and boats were ordered not to leave the country. For several days our communication with Joe was completely cut off, but then, finally, we received word he was safe. He had fled the country on a small fishing boat that eventually crossed paths with a Caribbean cruise ship and dropped him off at the next port. In a few months Haiti's political situation had stabilized and we sent a doctor back to the Pierre Payan clinic.

Over the years I made twenty-five to thirty trips to Haiti and never feared for my safety—except sometimes on the roads where speed limits were non-existent. On Saturdays, when my household tasks were finished, I enjoyed hiking up into the mountains with Mauresso, a Haitian friend. We would cross the highway, walk through the open market and follow a stream up through the mountain corridor. There are two Haitian sayings that I always thought about on these trips: "Behind every tree is a Haitian" and "Behind every mountain is another mountain." Both are true, but I'd suggest revising the second one, making it: "Behind every mountain is another mountain, higher and steeper." Many families lived along the stream since this was where they collected their drinking water, washed their clothes, and bathed. I learned from examinations at the clinic that the healthier people lived higher up the mountains—near the stream's source.

Haitians are among the most outgoing people I have ever met, and on these excursions I would be warmly greeted by basket-makers, bakers, woodworkers, and other craftspeople, as well as farmers and children. On our way up, we always passed by the voodoo doctor's home and his gathering place at the edge of the village, and then, after that, the homes were more scattered. One day when we had journeyed much further than usual, a woman hollered at us in Creole. "What did she say?" I asked Mauresso.

"She says she has never seen a *blanc* (white person) in this part of the mountain," he replied. We decided that maybe we had walked far enough for that day.

Occasionally, the mission held a medical clinic back in the mountains. Usually we only traveled as high as we could go with a four-wheel-drive Land Rover, but twice Erica Fast, a Canadian nurse, and I rode donkeys up to one of the mission churches to hold a clinic. This was hard riding, so I preferred walking except when we came to narrow places where one side of the path hugged the mountainside and the other dropped straight down, hundreds of feet. At these tricky places our guide said we were much safer riding the donkeys than trusting our own footwork.

Perhaps the most unfortunate trait of most small Indiana towns is their lack of racial and ethnic diversity. Because of this, townspeople often miss out on what I have found to be one of the most meaningful experiences in life—getting to know someone of a different culture. An exciting and unforeseen aspect of our Pierre Payan project was the way the Markle community got involved and thus had contact with many Haitians. Not long after the other doctors and I started flying down, individuals and work crews from Markle and other nearby towns started going with us. They formed friendships with the people of Pierre Payan as they participated in various projects, including constructing a shed, painting the clinic, adding a rubber bladder to the water tower, and installing a telephone system on the clinic compound. One on one, or with an interpreter, they talked with Haitians in the hospital and in the village, at the market, and at church.

Many of our nurses helped in the clinic, or they assisted at the Markle office by procuring and packing medicines and supplies. Young people got involved, too. For instance, in 1980 a freshman at Southern Wells high school, Lyle Towns, directed a project that collected over 340 pairs of eyeglasses for the Pierre Payan clinic. One year the town boxed up all its left-over t-shirts from past Wildcat Festivals and sent them to Haiti with Vic. Later I found it surreal to pass by Haitians in the market or in the clinic with t-shirts that displayed Markle's old schoolhouse or train depot, with slogans such as "Markle is for Me," "Those were the Days" or "History on the Wabash."

Since its inception, the Haitian clinic remained busy. Vic and two Haitian nurses might have set the record, though, when they saw two hundred and sixty patients in one day. In 1991 he and his second wife Donna, a nurse, decided they wanted to work full-time in Haiti. That September they left the Markle Medical Center and immediately started construction of a surgical addition to the Pierre Payen clinic, as well as overnight rooms. Gradually as the clinic expanded, staffed with more trained Haitian doctors, nurses, and technicians, Vic worked on designs for a full-fledged hospital.

In 2001, with financial support from the Markle Medical Center, the clinic's surgery and patient rooms were converted to an obstetrical delivery and overnight maternity ward and a new hospital opened across the road. This facility had a surgery suite, rooms for twenty-two patients, and an open courtyard Vic filled with bright tropical plants.

A SECOND OPINION

One night when my son Steve was only six years old, he started acting agitated and experiencing visual and auditory hallucinations. Lying on his bed, looking up, he saw the model train in the basement hanging upside down, as if the tracks were nailed to the ceiling. The engine and boxcars were circling 'round and 'round. Then he jumped up and shouted, "The police are coming! I hear the sirens. See—the police. They're coming for us. Laurel and Lynn, we gotta hide!" He dashed from room to room, crawling under beds and cowering in corners. Although Lee and Dawn's youngest children weren't there, he kept telling them to hide.

Earlier that day, before I went to work, I told Mary to give Steve Aveeno baths and liquid Benadryl. He had the chickenpox and was doing well except he kept scratching his sores. The Aveeno and Benadryl would alleviate the itching. When Mary asked how much Benadryl she should give, I said, "One teaspoon every four hours, but if you give him too much, he'll just get sleepy and that will be okay."

When I came home, Steve still seemed uncomfortable and was scratching his sores. So I gave him another dosage of Benadryl to quiet him down. As evening turned to night, Steve started hallucinating. I would hold him for a while until he agreed there were no police, but as soon as I let go, he'd jump down and start running and hiding.

When I was an intern at Lutheran Hospital I assisted in the care of a thirteen-year-old boy who was admitted with chickenpox encephalitis. That child died. I started imagining the worst. Did Steve have encephalitis or some other complication from chickenpox?

I needed another doctor's opinion so at about 11 p.m. I called up Neil Irick. Neil lived in an old farmhouse just across the gravel road from us and had recently joined the Markle Medical Center as its fourth doctor. He was a young physician, straight out of Indiana University School of Medicine, who had grown up in the small town of Buckeye, about ten miles south of Markle. Neil walked right over and after checking Steve asked what medicine we had been giving him. Mary said she had been spooning him Benadryl during the day, and I said I had given him several doses that evening. Neil quickly diagnosed Steve's behavior as a drug overdose. "Most people get sleepy from antihistamines," he said, "but a small percentage reacts in a totally opposite way. They become hyperactive and may even hallucinate."

Mary and I were relieved that all we needed to do was stop the flow of Benadryl. Towards morning, Steve settled down to sleep—and we did, too.

That night I was reminded of Vic's episode with his cat and also the words of Coach John Wooden: "It's what you learn after you know it all that counts."

MORE DOCTORS

When Lee and I moved into Dr. Wood's office on Morse Street, we never pictured our practice growing any larger than what two doctors could handle. But when Vic and then later Neil asked to join us, we were happy to gain their special skills. In fact, during the 1970s our practice was blessed with many new doctors we never recruited. They asked to join our practice because they knew someone on the staff or met us through a chance encounter. Although we didn't actively seek out these doctors, they seemed to always fulfill a certain need—providing expertise as a surgeon or OB-GYN or bringing a special interest in hospice care, anesthesiology, or pediatrics.

At first these doctors were all men. For years there just weren't as many women as men graduating from medical schools. I had a hundred and ninety-nine classmates at IU, but only four of them were female. Now the ratio is more balanced; in fact, IU medical school classes are over fifty-percent female. We were delighted in 1986 when Deborah Miller became the first female physician to join our practice. Later Dr. Tamara Dunmoyer brought her skills. Because she had grown up in Wells County, Tammy gained a devoted patient following from the start.

We made our employment agreements flexible so that if someone wanted to leave they could do so easily and on good terms. There were no penalties or restrictive covenants. There was also no pay scale until the 1980s. Doctors in other group practices advised us that pay should be linked to productivity, but Lee and I started out with a total sharing of income and expenses and this equal distribution of pay worked well for almost twenty years. In the 1980s, as some of the older physicians started slowing down and more specialists were hired, the doctors worked together to establish a fair pay scale.

Years before, in the early 1970s, our medical group had another important decision to make. The cost of malpractice insurance was doubling each year, but it did not seem right to charge our patients considerably higher prices to cover that increase. All of the doctors reached a consensus: we would go bare. We did not carry any malpractice insurance until 1975 when Governor Otis Bowen signed the Indiana Medical Malpractice Act which helped control insurance costs by capping the amount patients could collect in a lawsuit.

Having multiple doctors in our group meant we could learn from each other. Every Monday morning at 7 a.m., before we began rounds, all of the doctors in our practice met in the Wells Community Hospital lounge to converse over coffee. We met every week, even when our practice grew to ten doctors. We mostly talked about difficult cases we had at the hospital, but occasionally we also asked each other for advice about patients we were seeing for office visits. We often shared new information from medical journals, and when one of us attended a medical conference, we used this time to report on what we had learned about heart disease or neurology or maybe scheduling childhood immunizations. The social aspect of this meeting was important, too, because some of us might not see each other until the next Monday morning.

We would also have a business meeting every month or two, and during this time the doctors could talk about any problems in the practice before conflicts and tensions had a chance to build up. I believe these meetings were one reason why we all got along so well with each other. Physicians who joined us commented that they had never seen a group of doctors in which there was so little friction.

Our families socialized at an annual summer picnic hosted at one of the doctor's homes or at a park. We often met at Bluffton's Oubache State Park where we'd hoist a volleyball net, organize a scavenger hunt for the kids, and feast on Kentucky Fried Chicken along with homemade salads and desserts. In December we got together again, this time with all of our employees and their spouses for a festive Christmas party at a restaurant or catering hall. As president of the Markle Medical Center, my self-imposed duty each year was introducing all of the staff and their spouses and saying something personal about each one, all without notes. On our fortieth anniversary, when the staff had reached sixty, it meant I needed to recognize almost one hundred and twenty people and know their names. The pressure was on, but I succeeded. The entertainment for our Christmas parties was always volunteered (or pulled) from our own ranks. One of my favorite memories is when the doctors formed an angelic choir, garbed in white lab coats.

In 1973, with the Markle Medical Center attracting more patients and doctors, we opened a Bluffton office next to the Wells Community Hospital. Two years later we sold the Morse Street office to a dentist and built a larger facility at the edge of town. In 1986 we opened a third office in Warren, a small town about twelve miles from Markle. This move seemed to make sense since our practice already included many Warren residents and for fourteen years we had been sending a doctor to the Warren Memorial Methodist Home (now the Heritage Village Retirement Center) for a half day, five days a week.

By its fortieth anniversary, Markle Medical Center included ten doctors, three mid-levels, and a family counselor. Our doctors served three offices and twelve nursing homes. We had enough staff to provide assistance at health fairs, Bluffton's Panos Free Clinic, migrant medical clinics, drug and sex education programs, high school athletic events, and the Wells County Jail.

As the Markle Medical Center grew in size, it was important to Lee and me that it maintain its family-like atmosphere. When we opened our office, we were about the same age as most of our staff, and we all got along well, almost as if we were sisters and brothers. To keep that friendly, relaxed atmosphere, we knew it was essential to treat each member of our team with respect, whether he or she was a janitor, a nurse, or a doctor. This respect involved trust. Lee and I tried not to look over anyone's shoulder as a "boss," but to allow each staff member to use their best judgment.

During those years I only received two letters from employees with complaints that were critical of our operation. One was from a nurse's husband who said his wife did not feel we were treating her fairly and the other from a doctor's wife. I met privately with these people and listened to their grievances. In both cases the problems were resolved and the nurse and the doctor continued with us for many more years.

When it was just Lee and me, we saw patients on a rotating basis, so we knew all of our patients well. But as the practice added more doctors and patients, this was no longer feasible. Instead, doctors saw their own patients and each nurse was assigned to a particular doctor so she could also know her patients' histories. The nurses I worked with the longest were Janet Hines and Sheila Kracium. After a while these nurses knew me and our patients so well that they became adept at anticipating my instructions. They'd wait for me to give the go ahead, but their own readiness saved a lot of time.

As a group, our doctors represented a wide range of personality types, from gregarious to quiet; from jokester to the philosophical; from intense to laid-back. If patients didn't feel comfortable with one type of doctor, they could try another. The diversity of our doctors was embodied by the variety of their interests. Some of us shared similar hobbies, but on the whole our outside activities covered a wide gamut. For instance, John Wilson and David Brown were accomplished pianists who played for their patients in nursing homes and enlivened our Christmas parties with their duets. While Dave had a poor opinion of felines (he was so allergic to them that he refused to go on a house call to any home with a cat), Deb Miller had room in her car for all animals, regardless of species. We never knew what orphaned or injured creature she might carry to the office. Once she brought in a nest of wild baby rabbits she fed with an eye dropper each hour. She managed to slip other wild animals through our back door, but we turned the dead bolt when she pulled an injured skunk from her trunk. Even the vet wouldn't let her bring that patient into his office.

Vic and I also enjoyed caring for animals, and we both found yard work a pleasurable activity. But Vic took yard work to a whole new level. He built his own greenhouse and had an extensive knowledge of plants, as well as an artistic eye for landscaping. He and Marcelo Gavilanez, our OB-GYN, were the creative writers in our group, but Vic preferred plotting science fiction stories while Marcelo composed poetry. Marcelo, who was born in Ecuador, was fluent in Spanish and devoted many volunteer hours to treating Hispanic migrant workers and their children who worked on tomato farms in Wells and Jay counties. Joe Greene had an obsession with trains. He rode them, collected them, and had models coursing on tracks in his house. Lloyd Williams was by far our best golfer. Besides being good at any sport, from baseball to golf, Lee had skill as an artist. He painted landscapes, mostly on canvas, but because he was inventive, he sometimes painted on other things as well—even the creamy side of the turkey tail tree fungi that grew in our woods.

Despite their varied interests and talents, all of the doctors had two things in common: they were active in a local church community and they loved popcorn. The more doctors we brought in, the more the Markle Medical Center smelled like a movie theatre and less like an office.

GERIATRICS

In my early years at Markle, I was a doctor of many trades, enjoying all areas of medical practice. In fact, I had pursued general practice because I was fascinated by every specialized area in medical school and didn't want to limit myself to just one. I found pleasure in delivering babies and then caring for the mother and infant. I liked fixing simple fractures and dislocations. I gave anesthesia when surgeries were in the early morning before office hours. I performed surgeries for hernias, appendectomies, caesarians, tonsillectomies, and adenoidectomies and assisted with more complicated operations.

But as time passed and Vic joined our practice, I was happy to give up surgeries and didn't mind just assisting with C-sections. I took as much satisfaction in watching a patient get well with someone else performing the operation. I had always sort of struggled with surgery, and Vic made it look easy; surgery just came naturally for him. He changed our post-op care as patients started going home in a third of the time they did with me or the specialists we used.

When Marcelo Gavelanez, an obstetrician, joined us, I had no problem letting him get up in the middle of the night to deliver a baby. As other young doctors joined, I let some of them care for the babies and younger children.

Dr. David Meek had special interest and skills in anesthesia, so I eventually asked him to take over my responsibilities in that area. Now I no longer needed to keep up on new specialized drugs and procedures related to that area of medicine.

In 1990 I took leadership in setting up the first outpatient hospice organization in our area, a program that involved nurses, nursing aids, chaplains, volunteers, and other ancillary personnel. I found it rewarding to supervise a program that allowed the terminally ill to remain at home with their families, but when Dr. Bernhard Wiebe joined our practice, he was keenly interested in end-of-life situations, so I turned over the directorship of our hospice program to him and was glad to back him up when he wasn't available. Bernie expanded our hospice program to more counties, with increased services and personnel.

By the time I was fifty-five, my practiced had changed significantly. I saw only adult patients with chronic diseases and many elderly patients. I spent time in nursing homes, rather than neonatal units or surgery rooms. I especially enjoyed my older patients who I had seen for many years and whose relatives and family history I knew. We spent so much time visiting that sometimes these older patients would call up to reschedule their appointments, saying, "I don't feel good enough to see the doctor today." Many of these patients had life experiences I found fascinating. For instance, Daniel Michaels would talk with me about his WWI experiences when he served with the 414th Erie Telegraph Battalion. Dan, who enlisted in 1917 when he was twenty-one, had the distinction of being one of the last three living Wells County veterans from that war. He died in 1998 at age one hundred and one.

Harvey Hite was another older patient with many interesting stories. He had lived in three different centuries. Born in 1897, Harvey could remember when the land surrounding Markle and Warren was mostly covered by trees as big around as his kitchen table. He could recall the oil boom of the turn of the century when pumping stations dotted the countryside. When the Depression hit in 1929, he could recall the day he only had a quarter to his name. But what Harvey liked best to talk about were his years of farming and the vegetable gardens he planted. When I made house calls to his apartment in Warren, he would say, "I wish I could have me a little garden and a goat for milk. If I had just a piece of land the size of this room, I could feed a big family."

Harvey drove his car until he was ninety-nine years old and then the optometrist said his eyesight was impaired to the point he shouldn't drive anymore. When he was a hundred and three years old, laser surgery corrected his vision and he asked me, "How about if I go back to driving a car again? Since I had my eye surgery, I can see as well as I ever could."

I told him, "Your eyesight may be okay now, but your reflexes are slower. Don't you think it might be better if you don't buy another car?" He pondered that for a while and then replied, "I think you're right. I shouldn't drive."

Harvey kept busy, though, often checking on the younger women in his apartment house—women in their 80s and 90s—to make sure they were okay. He'd carry their groceries and fix things for them.

When I retired, Harvey Hite was a hundred and eight years old, still living by himself and still helping his neighbors. "God is the reason I'm standing here," he'd say. "God is in the good air we breathe. We can't get away from God. God is in us." Before he died on February 26, 2008 at the age of a hundred and ten years, he was the oldest man in

Indiana. He told me the worst part of getting old was having those close to you leave you: "All my old friends have passed away and my son died young—at the age of eighty-five."

Looking out for less fortunate neighbors was an old habit of Harvey's and part of the rural culture he grew up in. Over the years I saw neighbor helping neighbor when a farmer lost his hand in a corn picker, when one fell off a silo, when a young farmer was stricken with Lou Gehrig's Disease and another with Multiple Sclerosis. I also saw neighbors coming to the rescue when my older patients needed help managing their money, figuring out how to rotate their crops, or recuperating from an illness or injury. They would step up to help these older people even if it cost them some financial loss. Frequently the help came in such a discrete method that others in the community were not even aware of it.

One of my older patients, a bachelor farmer who valued his independence, had a strong network of neighbors who looked out for him. He suffered some of the symptoms of aging, like memory loss, but neighbors helped him with his farming and brought him meals. One Saturday morning, however, this older farmer decided on the spur of the moment to drive to Cincinnati by himself and didn't tell anyone. That was a mistake. I received a call on Sunday evening from one of his neighbors saying I needed to see my patient right away, as he had been badly beaten.

This older man was still trembling when I arrived and had many superficial cuts and deep bruises. He was also dehydrated and said he hadn't eaten for two days. He kept mumbling, "I was lost" and "I thought they were going to kill me." Gradually, he found the words to tell us what had happened. After he arrived in Cincinnati, he had gotten lost and several young men stopped his car, demanding that he hand over his key or they would kill him. He obliged, but then they beat him and shut him inside the trunk. They drove around the city for the rest of that afternoon and night. On Sunday morning they finally opened the trunk and then walked away, laughing. My patient didn't know where he was, but he somehow found his way out of the city and back to his neighbor who cared for him as he recuperated.

Time after time, I was struck by the resilience of my older patients, many of them farmers and farm wives who had survived the Depression, had fought in a war or watched loved ones go off to a war, had seen hometowns slip from thriving commercial centers to ghost towns, had watched their farmland flooded to make a reservoir, had learned to adapt to a host of technological and cultural changes, and had survived diseases and accidents. I concur with Scott Russell Sanders in his memoir, *A Private History of Awe*, when he says, "What's remarkable about old age is not that we wear out but that we last so long in the grip of gravity."

My patient Elsie Hart, a farmer and homemaker, was one such resilient woman. Born in 1888, she was seventy-six when we moved to Markle, but so healthy that I seldom saw her for health issues. I mostly grew to know her through attending the same church. Elsie's husband died when her two sons, Joseph and Frank, were still young, but she continued farming by herself. During the Depression, she managed to hold on to her farm through her strong determination, the help of her teenaged sons, and the kindness of neighboring farmers. Later, Frank left the farm to fight in WWII. Both sons attended our church and died almost two decades before Elsie did.

When Elsie was almost a hundred years old, Mary asked her secret for good health and longevity. She said it was relaxing in a hot bath every night. Several other factors might have also helped: Elsie never smoked; had a history of physical activity; was part of caring community; and was blessed with two daughters-in-law, Norma and Erma, who always looked out for her.

I know of another resilient and remarkable woman who grew up near Markle and lived to an advanced old age—one hundred and five years old. *Kilsoquah*, whose Miami name means "Sun-Woman," was the granddaughter of the famous Miami war chief Little Turtle and second cousin to Chief Peshewa who owned land in and around what is now Markle. She grew up in the village just south of the town, but sources disagree as to whether that was her birthplace. Some say she was born at the Forks of the Wabash, three miles west of Huntington, but in 1906 when asked where she was born, she told S. P. Kaler and R.H. Maring, "near Markle, in Huntington County."

In the last years of his life, Little Turtle would travel from the home of his adopted son, William Wells, near Fort Wayne to visit Kilsoquah and her family. I would guess that on one of these trips he inoculated Kilsoquah against the deadly smallpox virus. Little Turtle asked a surgeon in Fort Wayne to teach him how to give inoculations of Edward Jenner's new vaccine so he could vaccinate the children in his village. Little Turtle died in 1812 from what was then diagnosed as gout, later Bright's Disease, and now termed nephritis, but before he passed away, I feel certain that he would have inoculated his granddaughter.

Kilsoquah said her childhood was a happy one, as she was born "during the Great Spirit's cheerful smile," when "the wild woods were full of flowers and the wild berries near at hand." Later, however, she had to contend with many losses. Her first and second husbands both died as young men from illnesses. Four of her six children died in infancy. By the time of the Miami Removal in 1846, Kilsoquah lived on a land grant about ten miles from Markle near the current town of Roanoke. Like other Miami who were related to tribal leaders, she was allowed to stay in Indiana, but she would have watched sadly as many of her friends were forced to leave for Kansas.

Accounts of the Miami Removal describe the tribal members' anguish at leaving, how they clutched handfuls of earth from their ancestors' graves. Matilda Roush, a white settler who grew up two miles west of Markle, was an eyewitness and said that one Miami woman was so overcome with grief that she was unable to stand up and had to be carried to a wagon. Her daughter had died a few weeks earlier, and she could not bear to leave her grave in the burial ground just south of Markle.

Not only was Kilsoquah stranded without a local tribal community, but many of the wild animals she had revered disappeared, too. She saw the forest cut down, the wetlands drained. Her landholding of three hundred and twenty acres dwindled to forty. Her son's dislike of farming may have had something to do with that, but there were other factors, too. In an affidavit, Dr. Perry G. Moore mentions meeting Kilsoquah at the Wabash courthouse in 1887, where she was defending the title of her home against a man from Huntington.

By all accounts, Kilsoquah held on to the old ways. When the weather was warm, she liked to camp outside and did that each summer until she was one hundred and three years old and her worn tent fell apart. She smoked tobacco in a corn cob pipe and always wore calico dresses, two gold rings, and a red scarf. She pieced bright diamond shapes and quilted them into star-patterned quilts. She kept her Miami language, communicating with whites either through sign language or through her son. She spoke only a few dozen words of English but those who interviewed her noticed that her comprehension was keen.

Over the years Kilsoquah became good friends with a Roanoke physician—Dr. Sylvanius Koontz. The doctor asked her questions about Miami history and perhaps also inquired about her knowledge of tribal medicine. In *Indiana Magazine of History*, Ansel A. Richards mentions that Kilsoquah once cured his father when in boyhood he was bitten by a snake. Dr. Koontz gave Kilsoquah tobacco in exchange for her stories, and she gave him gifts, as well, including a miniature canoe she whittled herself. Dr. Koontz helped her reestablish contact with her daughter in Oklahoma and upon her request removed the remains of her husband from an unmarked gravesite so that when she died, they could be buried together.

By the turn of the century, Huntington County residents called Kilsoquah, *The Last Miami Princess*. On July 4, 1910, when she was a hundred years old, Roanoke honored her with a celebration that attracted ten thousand visitors. That parade was Kilsoquah's last public appearance in

Huntington County. In her final years rheumatism restricted her movements. She mostly moved between her bed and a chair cut from a barrel. She loved to quilt, but finally had to give that up when her vision failed — probably due to cataracts.

But Kilsoquah's mind remained sharp. People who interviewed her were impressed by how accurately she recalled details from her grandfather's battles, dates related to family history, and who was related to whom. Surely she must have remembered the dances at the confluence of the Rock Creek and Wabash, of those years when passenger pigeons flew in such numbers their flight darkened the sky. Did she take note in 1914 when the last passenger pigeon — Martha — died in a cage in the Cincinnati Zoo?

The public statement that Kilsoquah gave on July 4, 1910 begins with "My people are gone, those I knew are dead." Then she goes on to list all of the "marvelous" signs of progress she has seen — "the old canal, then the railroad, then the interurban and now the automobile." She says these changes were "wrought" and "wrought well" by "the hand of the Great Maker himself." But Kilsoquah saw her people taken away by canal boats. A train carried her daughter Mary from her. She never rode the interurban or owned an automobile. For her the parade of progress would have felt more like a procession of losses. Was her use of inflated language meant to convey a note of irony?

After all, this was the granddaughter of Little Turtle, a brilliant orator and military strategist. This was the cousin of Chief Peshewa, an astute negotiator. This was Kilsoquah — "Sun Woman" — who said her name meant "Setting Sun."

ALZHEIMER'S

The man is elderly but well-dressed. When we shake hands, he has a blank expression and empty eyes. Immediately, he starts pacing the room, sometimes approaching to mutter a few scrambled phrases that seem to mean something to him but that I can't interpret. His wife encourages him to sit down, and he does for a few seconds and then stands up to resume his pacing.

I go to him and put my hand on his thin shoulder: "Hello, Dad. I'm Gerald, your son. I came to visit. How are you feeling?"

He looks me over closely, mumbles a few more phrases, and then walks away. I want to think that he recognizes me, but nothing indicates he does.

My father, Perry, had late-onset Alzheimer's disease as did his father and several of his siblings. He lived to the age of eighty-seven, and except for the dementia which affected him the last five to six years of his life, was always in good health. For over fifty years, he taught school, beginning in a one-room schoolhouse in Michigan when he was only seventeen. Later, he taught seventh and eighth grades at Honeyville School in LaGrange County before becoming a history teacher and the grade school and high school principal at Shipshewana. In 1955 he began teaching full-time at Goshen College in its teacher-training program. He also taught one year in a teacher-training school in Kenya and three years at Rosslyn Academy in Nairobi. For two of those years, Dad served as Rosslyn's principal.

Dad was always a teacher at heart and proud that his classroom students included three generations of his family:

his wife, children, and oldest grandchild, Shari. Even after retirement, he kept teaching. When he was eighty-one, the *Goshen News* carried a photo of him with a sixty-year-old gentleman at McDonald's. The man was quoted as saying, "I just wanted to be able to read the morning newspaper, and now I can, thanks to Mr. Miller."

After my father died, my mother, Lucile, developed Alzheimer's and succumbed to it at age ninety-two. Mom had been a teacher, too, working in the elementary grades at Shipshewana and Goshen and also teaching with Dad in Kenya. She cared for him in their home, up to the last week before he died. When we visited her in the Alzheimer's unit at her nursing home, she'd hold our hand as we walked down the hallways or through the patio garden. Sometimes she'd invite us to stay until her husband arrived home for dinner.

It seems like I've always had an interest in those patients with dementia and maybe that interest started in the 1950s when my grandfather suffered with senility. He became so violent with his family who took turns caring for him that he had to be placed in a nursing home. The staff tied him down to restrain him, which only made him more agitated and restless. Dad would come home crying after his visits and worried that when he grew old he might become violent, too. For someone as even-tempered as my father, this was a hard concern to handle. Dad was so amiable that when as a young man he fell beneath the uninhibited scissors of a drunken barber who kept trimming upward, closer and closer to the top of his head, he didn't complain. Afterward, he just paid the bill and parted his hair straight down the middle, like

Alfalfa's on *The Little Rascals*. Dad decided he liked his new center part and never went back to the side option.

When I graduated from medical school, Alzheimer's disease was thought to affect only people under sixty-five; those older who had memory loss were diagnosed with age-related senility. So the first patient I identified with Alzheimer's was a woman in her fifties. She was single and worked at General Electric in Fort Wayne. Her family didn't like my diagnosis and took her to another doctor who said he could cure her. After two months, when she didn't improve and actually grew worse, he sent her to the Richmond Mental Hospital where she died two weeks later.

Now we know that Alzheimer's can affect those over sixty-five in the same ways that it affects those younger. In fact, the incidence of Alzheimer's keeps increasing with age. During the last fifteen years of my practice, I saw many older patients with Alzheimer's and found it rewarding to work with these patients and their families. As family members became aware of the problems associated with the disease and its progression, we set up support groups in Bluffton, Warren, and Markle. These were usually in nursing or retirement homes and in churches. We discussed how family members can manage to keep the patient safely at home for a longer period of time and without becoming burned out.

Of course it was sad to watch patients with whom I'd had a close relationship throughout the years succumb to dementia. In some respects it's like watching a busy main street lose its tenants, to see boarded windows where colorful displays once were. Those without family members in the area had the most difficult problems. One Markle woman was in her early eighties and living by herself when it grew increasingly apparent that she was becoming confused. She started repeating herself and asking others to help her with simple household tasks. She wouldn't admit that she had any difficulties and would get irritated when I suggested that maybe she needed to stay at the Markle Health Care Center where her husband was residing. One day I noticed her car had many fender dents and a scrape along the side. I spoke to our local policeman and garage mechanics who all told me that she should not be driving. Sometimes she drove on the wrong side of the street, and everyone was learning to watch out for her unpredictable sedan.

When I spoke with my patient, she said, "I'm not having any accidents. It's just that other people drive into my car when it's parked downtown. I can drive as well as I ever could. People are just picking on me."

The mechanics told me they had tried disconnecting her battery so she couldn't drive, but someone trying to be helpful always connected it back again. I called my patient's daughter in California, and she said she'd come and take care of the situation. But she also found her mother very difficult to manage. She went to the license branch in Huntington to see if it would take away her mother's license, but she was told, "Because your mother has never had a traffic ticket or accident report, we can't deny her driving privileges without her permission." The local police never ticketed this woman—they just drove her home. The only way we could have her license taken from her was if her daughter took her to court.

Instead, the daughter had the car disabled to the point that it could not be easily fixed and then told her mother that she couldn't afford to buy a new one. She convinced her mother to move into the nursing home because her husband needed her there.

Many of my Alzheimer patients were competent in regards to following the rules of the road because they had been at the wheel for so long they simply drove by habit. They'd have more problems with getting lost. One man came up missing after he set out to drive four miles to the Pizza Hut in Bluffton for a carry-out. The State Police called the Medical Center about noon the next day when they found him stopped south of Indianapolis at a highway construction zone, not knowing what to do. One patient was discovered in Illinois after she stopped to buy gas but had no money because she'd forgotten her purse.

Another Markle woman turned up just east of Chicago. Late one Sunday evening a truck driver called from a rest stop on the toll road to say a car started following his semi-truck on Interstate 69, north of Markle, and had followed him all the way onto the toll road, always tagging closely behind. When he pulled off at the rest stop, the driver pulled off, too. She told him she was on the way home from church and that she lived only a few houses away. Several members of her church drove up to Chicago to pick her up and return her home. Since she had no children, we made arrangements for her to be admitted to the Alzheimer unit in our local nursing home.

Significant gains have been made since my grandfather was moved to a nursing home. Medicines now help control the agitation and restlessness. Healthcare providers have humane and helpful ways for dementia patients to safely stay as active as possible at home or in a nursing facility. The

Alzheimer wing at the Markle nursing home plans a number of recreational activities for their patients. Mary enjoyed going to that unit to sing with the residents because they'd belt out without reserve, taking great pleasure in the old songs. She said the regular residents in the open lounge area sang with much less vigor, too self-conscious to sing out.

But despite the progress in our care of Alzheimer patients, we don't have a cure and the prospect of memory loss is frightening. Every day I work at least one Sudoku puzzle, not just because I enjoy the game, but also because the American Alzheimer's Association has endorsed it as an activity that might help decrease the risk of dementia. I work the puzzles in pen so that I don't go back to erase. Right now I work the four and five starred puzzles, but if I slip down to the next level, I know I'll start getting worried. I also try to keep my brain healthy by reading and writing and guessing the answers on quiz shows like Jeopardy. It takes me a little longer now to think of the answers, but that's normal for someone my age. As people get older, mental responses slow down. The information is still there—it just takes longer to recall it.

What's most worrisome about Alzheimer's and other forms of memory loss is the forfeiture of connection it entails. You no longer feel connected to beloved people and places and events. You are cut-off from your own life story.

Towns can have memory loss, too. A town can forget its distinctive stories, history, and traditions—its identity. It can fail to recall what ties it to a particular geographical area and to particular people and other living creatures. In that case, important connections that nourish understanding and create a healthy community are weakened or lost.

The film director John Huston once said, "You walk through a series of arches, so to speak, and then, presently, at the end of a corridor, a door opens and you see backward through time, and you feel the flow of time, and realize you are only part of a great nameless procession."

For me, that great procession is not nameless—at least not yet. I walk in the Wildcat Parade with others I have known—Randols and Mossburgs, Kinzers and Caleys—down Clark Street beneath the old, arching boughs of maples. At the bottom of the hill we round the corner, turning east on Morse Street. When I look backward through time, I see those who have come before me; I feel the flow of the river.

EPILOGUE

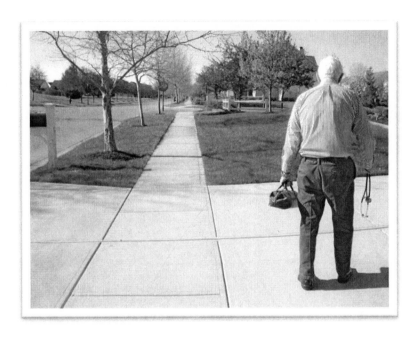

GOING BACK

Nine years ago Mary and I sold our house in the woods and moved ninety miles south to Westfield, Indiana where two of our three children, Shari and Stephen, live. We mostly made the move in order to be closer to our children and grandchildren but also because Mary believed, with good reason, that, unless we moved away, I would never be able to retire, to put away my medical bag and hang up my stethoscope.

But now we live in a suburban community north of Indianapolis where the traffic is congested and the only way we interact with our neighbors is with a wave as they pull in and out of their driveways. In Markle and other nearby communities, we always knew people when we went to the grocery store, bank, restaurants, and high school sporting events. Now we can shop at the Kroger store, no more than a half mile away, and not see a single person who looks familiar, except maybe the cashier or the person bagging groceries. We can attend an Indiana Pacers basketball game and be one of seventeen thousand in the stands and still not know anyone. Or we can go to a Colts game and be a stranger amid sixty-five thousand fans. We have a few festivals in our large subdivision, but when we attend, we don't recognize many people.

From Sunday to Sunday, we can be out and about and yet see no one we know. At least for two hours on Sunday we see familiar faces at the Mennonite church in Indianapolis. But because attendees come from all over the city and surrounding areas, we usually don't meet them during the week, unless they are in our small group. That group meets twice monthly and is our main source of friends.

Fortunately, I have remained healthy since my retirement. But now when I go to the doctor for my yearly appointment, I am the patient in the waiting room thumbing through magazines, the patient who would rather not step on the scales. When my doctor comes into the room, he's friendly, but he looks down at his hand-held computer as he talks with me, asking questions the screen tells him to ask. He seems to remember me, but I think that's because his computer reminds him. When the doctor orders lab work, I have to specifically request a copy of my report because, otherwise, I won't receive one. At Markle I always made sure my patients received their lab analysis, and I took time to educate them about what the words and numbers meant. That way they could be more knowledgeable about the status of their health.

Right now I am actually without a physician because mine has moved to another practice. His office is owned by a large hospital, and he's leaving to take a position at another hospital-owned practice. Mary has had two Westfield doctors, but both of them have moved away, too, and she is currently without a doctor. Shari's husband Chuck is also without a doctor because his has left for a town in northern Indiana. Since coming to Westfield thirteen years ago, Shari has had four different physicians because hers have moved away. Doctors in this suburban area don't seem to have much allegiance to the community. When another hospital-owned practice offers them a better salary or working conditions, they pick up and move on.

It appears there's an epidemic here, what Wendell Berry refers to as "one of the characteristic diseases of the twentieth century. . .the suspicion that [people] would be greatly improved if they were somewhere else." When doctors are infected, it's hard for them to build a strong rapport with their patients, to grasp their patients' family histories, and to appreciate how individual health is related to the health of the community.

Occasionally, Mary and I go back to Markle to visit friends or for special events. Last August we went back for the Wildcat Festival. A year earlier, the festival had dwindled to just an antique car show, but last year it made a triumphant rebound with the theme, "Rock Around the Clock: Remembering the 50s and 60s." We attended the Friday night pork chop dinner sponsored by the Markle Fire Department and then stayed for a swing dance sponsored by the Markle Medical Center (now owned by Lutheran Hospital as part of the Lutheran Health Network). Mary and I have never learned to dance—it was a forbidden pastime for Mennonites when we were growing up—but we listened to the music and had fun conversing with old friends. Saturday's events included the traditional Wildcat Parade led by the four grouches and a full schedule of activities that included a frog jumping contest, a cornhole tournament, sidewalk chalk art, and an exhibit of ice sculpture.

Returning for events at the Markle Church of the Brethren (now TurnPointe Community Church) and to the annual stockholders' meeting of Marklebank (now IAB Financial) gives us additional contact with old friends. Each year I appreciate being invited by Richard Randol and Dan Lipp to General Insurances' annual golf outing at Timber

Ridge in Bluffton. I never developed the skills it takes to be a good golfer, but playing as a partner with Don Hoopingarner and others always makes for a pleasant day and keeps me connected with the community.

All too often our return trips to Markle have been to the mortuary for the death of a friend. Sometimes those friends have been former office employees or their spouses. Those have been sad visits but mixed with joy and humor as they brought back memories of our close-knit staff.

In February of 2010 I returned to the Markle area to participate in a memorial service for Vic who died after an eight-month battle with pancreatic cancer. The weeks surrounding his death were very hard for me as we had worked so closely together at the office and in Haiti. At age seventy Vic still had so many interests—writing, working with stained glass, collecting tropical fish, gardening with his wife, Donna—and so many ambitious plans for the new hospital in Haiti that his death seemed untimely.

In fact, he died one month after an earthquake devastated Port-au-Prince and the surrounding countryside and just one day after returning from a final mission trip to visit the hospital and say good-bye to his Haitian colleagues. In the aftermath of the earthquake, Pierre Payen's hospital served as a center for many needing medical care. Teams of general surgeons, orthopedic surgeons, and a couple of neurosurgeons arrived to set fractures, perform amputations, and even do some spinal procedures. After Vic's death, the hospital underwent the renovations he had designed and was dedicated in 2012 as the Victor Binkley Hospital. Donna cut the ribbon.

Lee died at age eighty on June 24, 2012. For a year he had been having symptoms of a heart problem that included weakness and shortness of breath. He collapsed and passed away one morning after coming into the house from watering flowers. His funeral was held in the Markle Methodist Church, where the sanctuary was packed with community people.

I cannot remember any time in which Lee and I had an argument or disagreement that we didn't immediately resolve. I appreciated his quick humor, service ethic, and deep faith in God. He never expressed bitterness about the injury that cut short a professional baseball career. Instead, he considered it almost as a blessing, something that gave him perspective and showed him what was important in life—service to others. I am sure that, like Doc Graham in *Field of Dreams*, Lee had some regrets that he couldn't play the game he loved, but like the small-town doctor in the film, what he would have regretted more was not being a doctor.

One year Lee and I represented Markle's doctors from the past in the Wildcat Parade. We each glued on a black handlebar mustache and outfitted ourselves in string bow ties, bowler hats, and old-fashioned suits and vests. We borrowed walking sticks, and I brought out my antique medical bags. We took seats in a horse-pulled surrey and rode down Logan Street, the same street that brought us to town so many years earlier. Before the bridge, we turned east onto Morse Street and passed the dentist office where our medical center had once been and, before that, Dr. Woods' office with his name stenciled across the window.

As I get older, time itself seems to be a procession of people and events winding through streets, without beginning or end, like a dream we are all dreaming together. The author William Saroyan once asked, "Is the small town a place, truly, of the world, or is it no more than something out of a boy's dreaming? Out of his love of all things not of death made? All things somewhere beyond the dust, rust, and decay, beyond the top, beyond all sides, beyond bottom: outside, around, over, under, within?"

Is the town in this book, then, more dream than real? Is it the dream of an old man looking back? A wish against the rust and decay that claims so many small towns?

It might be a dream—but a dream can become real. Markle's wooded park with its quarry-carved pool, softball field, baseball diamond, tennis courts, picnic pavilions, and Boy Scout cabin began as a dream—one initiated in 1950 when the Markle Fish & Game Club purchased an abandoned quarry. In recent years, the town has added three smaller parks, too: Old Mill Park along the Wabash River, Veterans Park in downtown Markle, and Walkway Park at the eastern edge of town.

A town that can work together to create a swimming pool from a quarry, stage a play with a cast of forty-five men dressed up as women, elect its town grouches with good humor, produce a newspaper in which no one gets paid, recruit its own doctors, and take care of its members least able to care for themselves—a town such as that might well accomplish anything. With creativity and vigor, it can set its dreams into motion. The highways that have taken business away can also bring business back. The reservoir that diverts a river can also draw visitors to its preserved wildlife area and recreational lake.

Of course, there's no assurance that a dream will work out. The idea Lee and I and two Markle businessmen had to build and invest in a small neighborhood shopping mall like Yoder Shopping Center in my hometown of Shipshewana — one that had a grocery store, hardware store, and dry goods — never took off. We built it in the mid-70s, hoping that it would provide local jobs and that its convenience would keep business from traveling to Huntington, Bluffton, and Fort Wayne. But we couldn't match prices or choices with the discount stores at the edges of the other cities. Eventually, we sold the Country Square, but I thought at the time that it was a risk worth taking. Now when I go back I'm happy to see that the hardware store is still in business and that the rest of the building has been transformed by Connie Gast and Carol Hohe, identical twin sisters, into the thriving Markle Exit 86 Antique Mall — one of the town's most successful businesses.

"Our hopes and dreams are the bubbles of life we are blowing. They do not all have to break," said Eiffel Plasterer, a chemistry teacher, sorghum farmer, and Wizard of Bubbles who lived in Huntington County, not far from Markle. He helped my patient Elsie Hart keep her farm during the Depression by trading sorghum and cornmeal for her grain. For over sixty years, Eiffel entertained people with bubbles and shared his philosophy of life. He became nationally known when he appeared on the Dick Cavitt Show and when he encased David Letterman in one enormous bubble. "Bubbles will last if they do not break," Eiffel liked to say. His goal was to create the toughest bubble ever made. Before he died, he set a record when he kept one in a mason jar just one day shy of a year.

Dreamers are continually needed in any small-town council, club, or committee. They have a place in any parade that means to move forward. With a sense of the town's history behind them, they stride toward the future to create new job opportunities, attractive spaces, a sense of identity, and openness to diversity. If they have these things, small towns can lure their young people back. They can be the kind of vital, healthy community that's harder to achieve in suburbs and cities.

One of my dreams is that more young doctors will recognize the rewards of practicing medicine in a small town or rural community. They will see how meaningful it is to make their rounds in a place they feel rooted to, where their patients are their neighbors, where they can provide healthcare that's connected to the past, present, and future.

These doctors will know what the old string doctors knew—that human attention is healing. They will want to hear the whole story. They will listen with their hand off the doorknob.

ABOUT THE AUTHORS

Gerald L. Miller, M.D. was born in 1937, in Goshen, Indiana, and grew up on a farm near Shipshewana, in a Mennonite family with a strong lineage of teachers, farmers, and missionaries. During his high school years, he raised calves for 4-H, played guard for his school's basketball team, worked as school janitor, and painted houses and barns with his father. He also dated a classmate, Mary Mishler, whom he married while in his second year of premed at Goshen College.

After graduating from Indiana School of Medicine, Gerald set up a family practice with his medical partner, Dr. Lee Kinzer, in the small town of Markle, Indiana. For forty-two years, he worked in this largely rural area south of Fort Wayne. During this time, Gerald regularly made house calls to those unable to come to the office and developed community home health care and hospice services. To provide better emergency care for his patients, he helped his community develop the first rural EMT and paramedic services in Northeast Indiana.

From 1971-72, Gerald and Mary, along with their three children, Shari, Marlis, and Stephen, spent a year of service with Eastern Mennonite Mission Board in Somalia, East Africa. He recounts this year in his memoir, *A Hundred Camels: A Mission Doctor's Sojourn and Murder Trial in Somalia* (Cascadia, 2009). Over the course of thirty-two years, he also made twenty-five trips to Project Help in Haiti. There, with the effort of other doctors in his medical practice and support from the Church of God, he helped establish a medical clinic and then a hospital.

Since 2006, Gerald and Mary have been living in Westfield, Indiana, where Gerald spends time gardening, golfing, reading, playing card games, and attending his grandchildren's extracurricular activities. He and Mary enjoy traveling, often with friends from their church, First Mennonite of Indianapolis.

Gerald can be reached at drglmiller@gotown.net.

Shari Miller Wagner grew up near Markle, Indiana and is a 1976 graduate of Norwell High School. After majoring in English at Goshen College, Shari worked in Louisiana as a Mennonite volunteer for the Clifton-Choctaw, researching the tribe's history and tutoring the school children. Later, at Indiana University, she studied poetry in the MFA program where she met her husband Chuck Wagner, another student in the program. Over the years, Shari has taught creative writing in universities, elementary schools, community centers, libraries, veteran centers, and nursing homes. She has been an instructor with the Indiana Writers Center for the last eight years.

In addition to collaborating with her father on this book and a memoir about her family's year in Somalia, *A Hundred Camels*, Shari is the author of two volumes of poems: *The Harmonist at Nightfall* (Bottom Dog Press, 2013) and *Evening Chore* (Cascadia Publishing, Dreamseeker Books, 2005). Her poems have appeared in *The Writer's Almanac* with Garrison Keillor, Ted Koosier's *American Life in Poetry*, *The Christian Century*, *Shenandoah*, *North American Review*, and the anthologies, *Best American Non-required Reading, 2013* and *A cappella: Mennonite Voices in Poetry* (University of Iowa, 2004). Her personal essay about Somalia, "Camels, Cowries, & a Poem for Aisha" was co-winner of *Shenandoah's* The Carter Prize for the Essay.

While her mother, Mary Miller, was editor of the *Markle Times*, Shari traveled to Markle from Indianapolis to write feature articles about the older residents of her hometown community. She was struck, like her parents, by the resiliency, humor, and wisdom of these men and women and intrigued by their descriptions of Markle in the early twentieth century.

You can contact Shari through her Facebook page (www.facebook.com/pages/Shari-Wagner/386120974838870) or by emailing sharimwagner@aol.com.

THE MILLER FAMILY

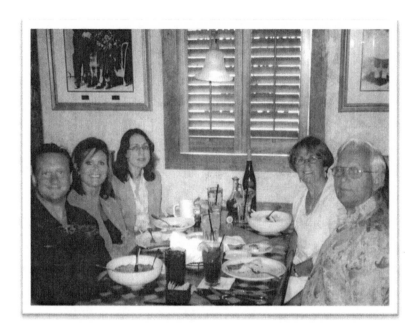

Stephen, Marlis, Shari, Mary, Gerald

CPSIA information can be obtained at www.ICGtesting.com
Printed in the USA
LVOW11s1603310815

452225LV00001B/161/P